The International Medical Graduate's Guide to
US Medicine & Residency Training

Patrick C. Alguire, MD, FACP • Gerald P. Whelan, MD, FACEP • Vijay Rajput, MD, FACP

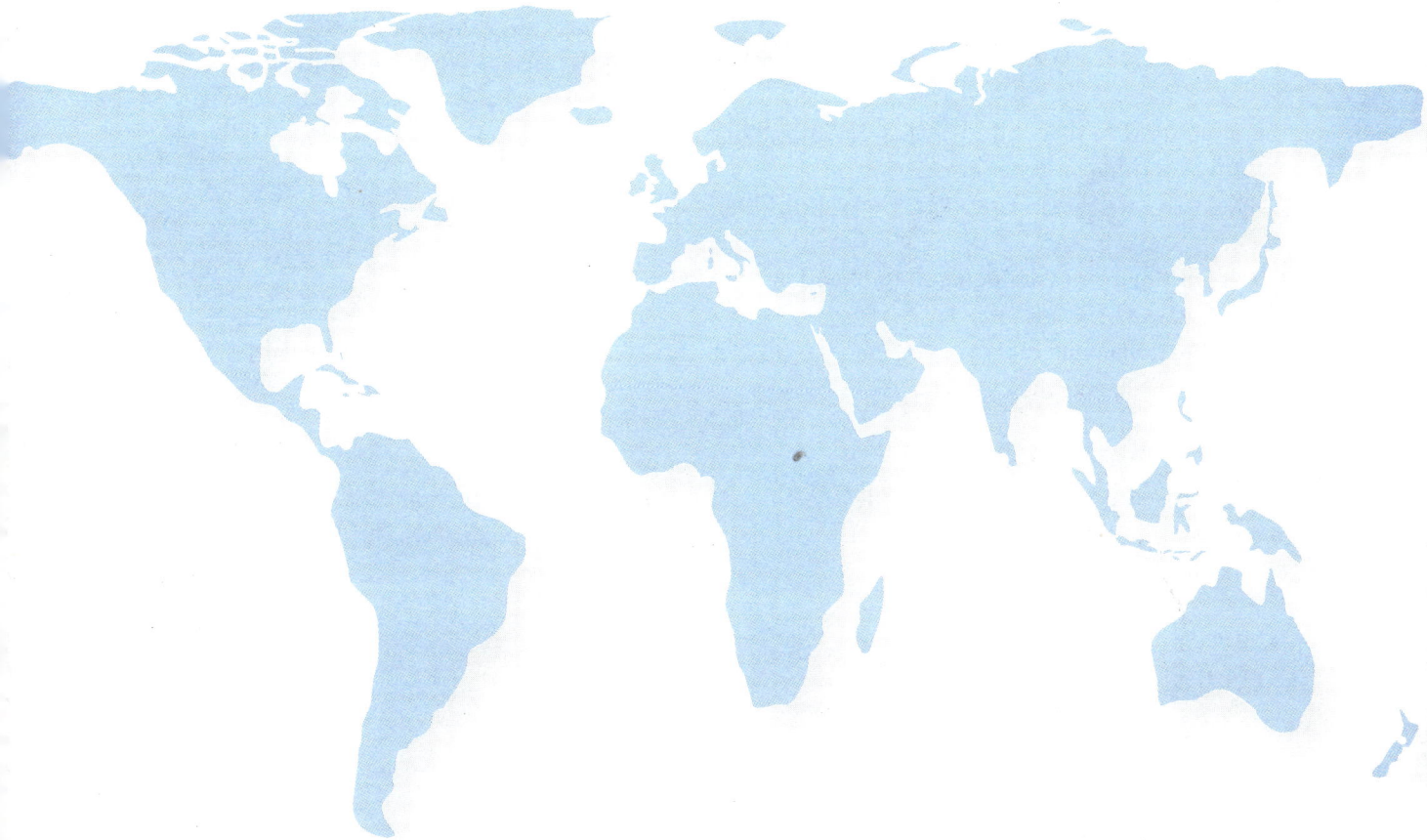

ACP®
PRESS

ECFMG®

Developed in collaboration with ECFMG

Associate Publisher and Manager, Books Publishing, Tom Hartman
Developmental Editor, Marla Sussman
Production Supervisor, Allan S. Kleinberg
Senior Editor, Karen C. Nolan
Editorial Coordinator, Angela Gabella
Marketing Associate, Caroline Hawkins
Cover Design, Lisa Torrieri
Interior Design, George W. Purvis IV
Indexer, Nelle Garrecht

Manufactured in the United States of America
Printing/binding by Versa Press
Composition by ATLIS Graphics, Gettysburg, Pennsylvania

Library of Congress Cataloging-in-Publication Data

The international medical graduate's guide to US medicine & residency training / edited by Patrick Alguire, Gerry P. Whelan, and Vijay Rajput.
    p. cm.
  ISBN 978-1-934465-08-0
1. Medicine--Study and teaching (Graduate)--United States.   2. Medical students, Foreign--United States.
3. Physicians, Foreign--United States.   I. Alguire, Patrick C. (Patrick Craig), 1950–   II. Whelan, Gerry P.
III. Rajput, Vijay.

  R840.I58 2008
  610.71'1--dc22   2008023588

09 10 11 12 13 / 10 9 8 7 6 5 4 3 2 1

Editors

Patrick C. Alguire, MD, FACP
Director, Education and Career Development
American College of Physicians
Philadelphia, Pennsylvania

Gerald P. Whelan, MD, FACEP
Adjunct Associate Professor of Emergency Medicine
Drexel University School of Medicine
Director, Acculturation Program
Educational Commission for Foreign Medical Graduates
Philadelphia, Pennsylvania

Vijay Rajput, MD, FACP
Associate Professor of Medicine
Program Director, Internal Medicine Residency
University of Medicine and Dentistry of New Jersey / Robert Wood Johnson Medical School
Cooper University Hospital
Camden, New Jersey

Contributors

Balu Athreya, MD
Division of Rheumatology
Alfred I. duPont Hospital for Children
Wilmington, Delaware

Nancy Calabretta, MS, MEd
University of Medicine and Dentistry of
    New Jersey
Camden County Library
Cooper University Hospital
Camden, New Jersey

Susan K. Cavanaugh, MS, MPH
Evidence-Based Medicine Librarian
University of Medicine and Dentistry of
    New Jersey
Camden Campus Library
Cooper University Hospital
Camden, New Jersey

Vani Dandolu, MD, MPH
Associate Professor, Obstetrics, Gynecology and
    Reproductive Sciences
Residency Program Director, Obstetrics,
    Gynecology and Reproductive Sciences
Associate Professor, Public Health (College of
    Health Professions)
Temple University Hospital
Philadelphia, Pennsylvania

Eleanor M. Fitzpatrick, MA
Manager, Exchange Visitor Sponsorship Program
Educational Commission for Foreign Medical
    Graduates
Philadelphia, Pennsylvania

Emily Hartsough
Medical Education Coordinator, Internal
    Medicine Residency Program
University of Medicine and Dentistry of New
    Jersey / Robert Wood Johnson Medical School
Cooper University Hospital
Camden, New Jersey

Anna Headly, MD, MFA
Division of Undergraduate Medical Education
    in Medicine
University of Medicine and Dentistry of New
    Jersey / Robert Wood Johnson Medical School
Cooper University Hospital
Camden, New Jersey

Barbara J. Hoekje, PhD
Director, English Language Center
Drexel University
Philadelphia, Pennsylvania

Anna M. Iacone
Manager, ERAS Support Services at ECFMG
Educational Commission for Foreign Medical
    Graduates
Philadelphia, Pennsylvania

Ami Sharad Joshi, DO, MBA
Assistant Professor of Medicine
Internal Medicine Hospitalist
Program Director for Fellowship in Advanced
    Hospital Medicine
University of Medicine and Dentistry of New
    Jersey / Robert Wood Johnson Medical School
Cooper University Hospital
Camden, New Jersey

Anuradha Lele Mookerjee, MD, MPH, FACP
Assistant Professor of Medicine
University of Medicine and Dentistry of New
    Jersey / Robert Wood Johnson Medical School
Cooper University Hospital
Camden, New Jersey

Barbara A. Porter, MD, MPH
Assistant Professor of Medicine
Deputy Director, Division of Undergraduate
    Medical Education in Medicine
Department of Internal Medicine
University of Medicine and Dentistry of New
    Jersey / Robert Wood Johnson Medical School
Cooper University Hospital
Camden, New Jersey

Christy A. Rentmeester, PhD
Assistant Professor, School of Medicine
Center for Health Policy and Ethics
Creighton University Medical Center
Omaha, Nebraska

Stephen S. Seeling, JD
Vice-President for Operations
Educational Commission for Foreign Medical
  Graduates
Philadelphia, Pennsylvania

Hiren Shingala, MD
Chief Resident, Internal Medicine Residency
  Program
University of Medicine and Dentistry of New
  Jersey / Robert Wood Johnson Medical School
Cooper University Hospital
Camden, New Jersey

Antoinette Spevetz, MD, FCCM, FACP
Associate Professor of Medicine
Associate Director, MSICU for Operations
Director, Intermediate Care Unit
Associate Director, Internal Medicine Residency
  Program
Section of Critical Care Medicine
Cooper University Hospital
Camden, New Jersey

Marta van Zanten, MEd
Research Associate
Foundation for Advancement of International
  Medical Education and Research
Philadelphia, Pennsylvania

Edward Viner, MD
Professor of Medicine
Senior Vice President for Affiliations and External
  Development
University of Medicine and Dentistry of New
  Jersey / Robert Wood Johnson Medical School
Cooper University Hospital
Camden, New Jersey

Tracy Wallowicz
Department of State Case Manager
Educational Commission for Foreign Medical
  Graduates
Philadelphia, Pennsylvania

Foreword

In recognition of the important role that international medical graduates (IMGs) play in health care in the United States, the Educational Commission for Foreign Medical Graduates (ECFMG) and the American College of Physicians (ACP) have collaborated to develop *The International Medical Graduate's Guide to US Medicine & Residency Training*, a unique resource for IMGs and for residency program staff involved in graduate medical education (GME). The authors and editors of this book have attempted to put into one resource information on all aspects of the processes by which IMGs can achieve ECFMG certification, secure positions in U.S. GME programs, obtain appropriate immigration status, understand and function within our unique medical education and health care delivery system, and settle in to working and living in America. The book not only brings together all relevant information from various sources but also presents it in a way that provides some context, practical advice, clarity, and easy accessibility.

Since its inception in 1956, ECFMG has provided the support for IMGs to obtain the necessary certification that would allow them to enter supervised programs accredited by the Accreditation Council for Graduate Medical Education (ACGME) in the United States. ECFMG's efforts have centered on access to the necessary examinations and verification of credentials documenting completion of acceptable undergraduate medical education. ECFMG has also had a long-standing commitment to providing information to IMGs and GME program staff regarding many other aspects of IMG transition and entry to American medicine, as well as the challenges of living and working in the United States. Recently, in recognition of the important role that IMGs play in American health care and the reality that that role will continue to be significant for the foreseeable future, ECFMG has increased its efforts to assist IMGs by creating a new Acculturation Program. Its goals are to develop and make available an array of resources for IMGs contemplating or in the process of pursuing entry to U.S. GME in order to facilitate their transition to American medical education, the American health care system, and American culture.

Founded in 1915, the American College of Physicians is the national organization for specialists and trainees in internal medicine and all its subspecialties. With approximately 125,000 members, ACP is the largest medical specialty organization in the United States. Since IMGs commonly choose careers in internal medicine and it subspecialties, this collaboration brings together two of the major medical education organizations in the United States with respect to IMGs and their unique needs and issues. However, because the issues faced by IMGs are certainly not unique to those planning to enter residency training in internal medicine, this book is equally well suited to provide information and guidance to IMGs intending to train, or currently training, in all disciplines of medicine.

While it is hoped that this volume will provide a central and comprehensive resource on all important issues, the reader should be aware that many of the issues addressed can be quite complex, that exceptions to rules may apply, and that requirements, regulations, and laws are constantly subject to change. As the transitioning process to training in the United States moves forward, it is therefore essential for IMGs to check with definitive sources for up-to-date information and instructions. These sources are the ECFMG, with respect to certification issues, the Exchange Visitor Sponsorship program, and ERAS support services; the NRMP, for issues relating to the residency match process; the U.S. Department of State, for visa issues; and, once a contract is in place for a residency position, the program director and staff of that GME program.

The logic of having ECFMG and ACP work together on helping IMGs with the acculturation process in residency training became apparent to both of us at a lunch meeting we had several years ago, when we recognized the common interests of ECFMG and ACP in helping IMGs transition to training in the United States. The two of us, speaking for ourselves as well as for the organizations we represent, are delighted to see this unique resource resulting from our collaboration. We feel privileged to be able to facilitate the entry of qualified IMGs to U.S. GME and the U.S. health care system. We appreciate the contributions IMGs make to improved patient care both here in the United States and in their home countries.

A work with such a broad scope inevitably may have shortcomings. We welcome constructive feedback that will guide future revisions and enhancements. The list of contributors is extensive, and we are grateful for all they have done to make this book as comprehensive as it is. Thanks are also due the many unnamed reviewers in both organizations who provided invaluable suggestions and comments.

Finally, we must compliment the editors—Drs Patrick Alguire, Gerald Whelan, and Vijay Rajput—for their outstanding job in transforming the idea of such a resource into the reality of the volume you hold in your hands. We sincerely hope *The International Medical Graduate's Guide to US Medicine & Residency Training* will meet your needs and prove invaluable to both IMGs and program directors.

James A. Hallock, MD
President and CEO
Educational Commission for Foreign Medical Graduates

Steven E. Weinberger, MD, FACP
Senior Vice President for Medical Education and Publishing
American College of Physicians

Contents

Foreword   vii
James A. Hallock and Steven E. Weinberger

Section I

Before Starting a Training Program

Chapter **1**   An Overview of Residency Training in the
United States   3
Gerald P. Whelan

Chapter **2**   Obtaining a Residency Position in the United States   11
Gerald P. Whelan, Stephen S. Seeling, and Vijay Rajput

Chapter **3**   Applying to Programs   25
Gerald P. Whelan, Anna M. Iacone, Vijay Rajput, Emily Hartsough,
Anna Headly, Patrick C. Alguire, and Barbara A. Porter

Chapter **4**   Transitioning to the United States   57
Eleanor M. Fitzpatrick and Tracy Wallowicz

Section II

Entering a Training Program

Chapter **5**   Language and Communication   69
Barbara J. Hoekje and Marta van Zanten

Chapter **6**   American Medical Culture   89
Gerald P. Whelan

Chapter **7**   Patient Care   95
Balu Athreya, Hiren Shingala, Vijay Rajput, Gerald P. Whelan,
Anuradha Lele Mookerjee, and Stephen S. Seeling

Chapter **8**   Understanding the American Medical System   133
Edward Viner, Ami Sharad Joshi, Barbara A. Porter, Vijay Rajput,
Patrick C. Alguire, Susan K. Cavanaugh, Nancy Calabretta, Antoinette
Spevetz, Christy A. Rentmeester, Vani Dandolu, and Gerald P. Whelan

Chapter **9**   Assessment, Feedback, Evaluation, Certification,
and Licensing   171
Patrick C. Alguire

Chapter **10**   Living in America: Popular Culture   187
Gerald P. Whelan

Appendices

A. Glossary of Frequently Used Terms, Abbreviations,
    and Acronyms   201
B. Internet Web Sites   204
C. References   208
D. Educational Commission for Foreign Medical Graduates
    (ECFMG) Resources   209
E. The ECFMG IMG Advisors Network (IAN)   210
F. Ethnic Medical Societies   213
G. A Patient's Bill of Rights   216

    Index   219

Additional resources are available at www.acponline.org/IMGguide.

Before Starting a Training Program

1 An Overview of Residency Training in the United States

Gerald P. Whelan, MD

Basic Requisites
4

Structure and Length of Graduate Medical Education Training
4

Teaching and Learning in Graduate Medical Education
4

Osteopathic Graduate Medical Education
6

International Medical Graduates in the United States
7

Trends, Numbers, Countries of Origin, and Disciplines   7

Career Paths   8

Basic Requisites

Graduate medical education (GME) in the United States is an integral part of both the medical education system and the health care delivery system. GME is that phase of medical education which occurs after an individual has completed all requirements and received a doctor of medicine (MD) degree or its equivalent (e.g., MBBS). Training is now concentrated in a particular area of medicine or surgery, generally referred to as a *specialty* or, for advanced training within a specialty, a *subspecialty* (often called a *superspecialty* in other countries). In this book, the term GME, unless otherwise specified, may refer to either specialty or subspecialty training.

Structure and Length of Graduate Medical Education Training

Basic training in a specialty generally requires a minimum of three years but, depending on the specialty, may be considerably longer. The academic year in almost all programs begins around July 1, although most programs require newly arriving residents to arrive earlier for orientation and processing.

GME programs in the United States are designed according to the principle of graduated responsibility. This means that as trainees progress successfully from year to year they are given increasing responsibility for patient care and exercise more and more autonomy in the management of their patients. Nevertheless, all residents in training work under the direction and supervision of attending physicians ("attendings"). These are senior physicians, generally having completed formal GME training in their specialty and having achieved certification in their specialties or subspecialties. Ideally they have some years of experience beyond their training. When working in programs associated with academic centers, they hold faculty positions (Assistant Professor, Associate Professor, Professor, etc.) and may be involved in clinical or other research and publication in addition to their teaching responsibilities. Some may be full-time, but others may hold adjunct or voluntary clinical positions with full-time practices outside of the GME program or institution. Most importantly, the attending physician has ultimate legal and ethical responsibility for the care provided by all physician trainees working under his or her supervision. As such, attendings have the final word on all patient management decisions and must be kept informed of all patient developments, progress, or complications in a timely manner.

Teaching and Learning in Graduate Medical Education

While attendings have responsibility for clinical teaching at the highest level, clinical teaching is in fact a shared responsibility of all physicians in a GME program. Senior residents are expected to teach junior residents and even beginning residents are expected to teach medical students and other medical and nursing staff and trainees.

The bulk of teaching and learning in GME programs in the United States is clinical in nature, meaning it is case-based (patient-based) and occurs on the wards and in the units, operating rooms, and clinics, where patient care is being delivered. One common method employed is that of "rounds," a term that comes from the practice of a group of doctors and students going around from patient to patient to assess their status, discuss diagnoses, and agree on treatment plans. These may be "work rounds," conducted by senior residents and those whom they are supervising, or they may be more formal attending or teaching rounds, conducted by the attending physician. In either case it is typical that the patient is "presented" by one of the physicians (often more junior) followed by an exchange of questions and answers and an often free-ranging discussion about individual patients, as well as more generic discussion about pathophysiology, pharmacology, diagnostics, etc. Residents are expected to be prepared with accurate and current information about their patients, as well as general knowledge commensurate with their level of training and experience. Active participation by all is encouraged and is in fact expected by attendings.

Teaching also occurs in structured didactic conferences and presentations, and residents and fellows are expected to read and learn on their own from other sources regarding their patients and their specialty. These resources are described more fully in the section on the Educational Process in Chapter 8.

Completion of a GME program is not necessarily required to obtain a license to practice medicine in the United States, but all states require completion of some portion of an accredited GME program for licensure (see section on USMLE in Chapter 2). For international medical graduates (IMGs), the GME requirement as a precondition for unrestricted licensure ranges from three years (30 states), to two years (19 states), down to only a single year in 3 jurisdictions.

Successful completion of a program accredited by the Accreditation Council for Graduate Medical Education (ACGME) qualifies a physician to sit for specialty certification examinations administered by the member boards of the American Board of Medical Specialties (ABMS). ABMS specialty certification is distinct from, and not required for, medical licensure; however, the vast majority of American physicians, including IMGs, have specialty certification. Those who do not may face restrictions in their practice options and may have difficulty obtaining hospital privileges. All ABMS specialty boards require participation in ongoing Maintenance of Certification (MOC) programs, which include periodic examinations.

GME also includes fellowship training. Fellows are physicians who have generally completed a basic residency and are pursuing more advanced and specialized training in limited areas of medicine or surgery, generally referred to as *subspecialties* (*superspecialties* in some countries). Duration of fellowship training varies by subspecialty; there is a one-year minimum, although most programs are longer. Many fellowships are accredited by the ACGME and can lead to further certification by an ABMS specialty board in the subspecialty. However, other fellowships, often more procedurally oriented, are not accredited by ACGME, and no additional certification results from completion of training. While IMGs training on visas are eligible to participate in ACGME-accredited fellowships, special inquiry should be made regarding eligibility to participate in non-accredited fellowships.

Although residents and fellows are physicians in training, they also provide a great deal of care for patients in the institutions in which they train and as such are employees of those institutions. However, they continue to be students, so they must balance their responsibilities to their education with their requirements to provide patient care services. The ACGME has general and special requirements that address the essential elements of the medical education program, as well as the clinical responsibilities that residents can be assigned. Residents are restricted to an average of 80 hours of clinical time per week, but because the 80 hours are averaged over a four-week period, there may be weeks when hours are slightly longer.

Institutions that offer GME programs must meet a number of general requirements regarding institutional support, resources, and working conditions for residents. Individual programs are then subject to more specific special requirements, which are developed and monitored by Residency Review Committees (RRCs) for each medical and surgical specialty. These requirements address resident educational and clinical experience, requisite faculty and supervision, and other particulars unique to each specialty. Programs periodically undergo site reviews by RRCs to determine if and for how long accreditation will be renewed. Programs that cannot retain accreditation cannot continue to function, and residents in a program that loses accreditation must seek positions elsewhere. Fortunately, this is an extremely rare occurrence.

ACGME specifies a number of core competencies that must be addressed in all GME programs and also specifies requirements for periodic evaluation and feedback to residents with advancement in a program contingent upon satisfactory performance (see Chapter 3). Most of these evaluations are based on direct observations by attending physicians and more senior residents, but some programs will also include input from nursing staff and others with whom residents interact. Programs may have a number of locally developed written or practical examinations as part of the of the evaluation process. Most programs also participate in annual "In-Training" examinations that are developed and administered by ABMS specialty boards or specialty societies. These are standardized national examinations and hence provide residents assessment of their knowledge with respect to their specialty not only relative to their peers in their own program but in relation to all residents in their specialty across the country.

Osteopathic Graduate Medical Education

Osteopathy is a uniquely American medical tradition that incorporates all of allopathic medicine (the traditional medicine practiced in the United States) but adds an emphasis on musculoskeletal manipulation. More information on the osteopathic tradition can be found online at www.do-online.org. Graduates of osteopathic medical schools receive a Doctor of Osteopathy (DO) degree rather than the Doctor of Medicine (MD) degree conferred on graduates of traditional medical schools. As such, osteopathy represents a parallel but considerably smaller medical tradition in the United States, although the structure and organization is quite similar to the allopathic tradition.

Osteopathic GME programs are accredited by the American Osteopathic Association (AOA) and are open only to graduates of osteopathic medical schools in the United States; they do not admit IMGs. However, because the number of graduates of U.S. osteopathic medical schools exceeds the number of available osteopathic GME positions, it is not uncommon for osteopathic graduates to seek entry into allopathic GME programs, and there are no barriers to their doing so. In that respect, osteopathic graduates are in competition with IMGs for entry into ACGME-accredited GME programs. It is also quite possible that IMGs entering U.S. GME programs may find themselves working with DOs and hence should be familiar with their credentials.

International Medical Graduates in the United States

TRENDS, NUMBERS, COUNTRIES OF ORIGIN, AND DISCIPLINES

IMGs from countries all around the world have sought and continue to seek entry into U.S. GME programs. In recent years, the Educational Commission for Foreign Medical Graduates (ECFMG) has received applications from medical students and physicians from over 200 countries. There are, however, some countries that consistently tend to produce more applicants than others. The ten countries from which the most applicants came in 2006 are shown in Table 1-1.

TABLE 1-1

Educational Commission for Foreign Medical Graduates (ECFMG) Applicants by Country of Medical School, 2006

Country of Medical School	ECFMG Applicants
India	3817
Pakistan	968
Dominica	713
Philippines	702
Grenada	671
Netherlands Antilles	572
China	501
Mexico	421
Cayman Islands	354
Egypt	344
Nigeria	344

IMGs have historically played a significant role in American medicine and continue to do so today. Currently, approximately one fourth of all physicians in GME programs are IMGs, and approximately one fourth of all physicians in practice in the United States are IMGs. These figures include physicians who are American citizens but who have completed medical school outside of the United States or Canada. Hence the percentage of physicians coming to the United States from other countries is somewhat less than one fourth, but it is still quite significant.

IMGs have pursued training and done quite well in literally all medical specialties and subspecialties. Historically, there are some specialties wherein they have been more prevalent. These specialties show some tendency to change from year to year but consistently include most of the primary care specialties. Table 1-2 shows the distribution of

TABLE 1-2

International Medical Graduate (IMG) Entry-Level Residents by Specialty, 2006

Specialty	IMG Residents
Internal medicine	3270
Family medicine	1234
Pediatrics	582
General surgery	464
Psychiatry	346
Ob-Gyn	228
Pathology	174

IMG residents in entry-level positions (first year of GME) among the seven specialties in which they were most prevalent in 2006.

CAREER PATHS

Upon completion of an ACGME-accredited program (residency and/or fellowship) and especially upon achieving specialty and/or subspecialty board certification by an ABMS member board, IMGs have exactly the same career options as do graduates of U.S. medical schools. Specifically, there are no positions within American medicine wherein an otherwise qualified physician can be denied entry simply on the basis of his or her being an IMG. Hence all career options are open to IMGs, and IMGs have pursued them all. IMGs are in academics, in research, in private practice, in hospitals and institutions, and in government and military positions, as well as in medical administration and academic leadership roles.

In practice, however, IMGs tend to follow the distribution of their residency training, so many commit to primary care, often in parts of the country that are medically underserved such as rural areas, inner city areas, or areas where there is a high concentration of immigrant patients. Some IMGs develop practices that are very much focused on patients of their own ethnicity, but others choose to pursue a more typically diverse practice.

Immigration status has a direct effect on the career options of an IMG. Specifically, on completion of training in an accredited program (residency or fellowship) or seven years after initial entry on the J-1 visa (whichever occurs first), IMGs on J-1 Exchange Visitor visas are legally bound to return to their home country for a minimum of two years before applying for re-entry into the United States. However, this requirement may be waived under some circumstances. Most commonly, waivers are available to an IMG who accepts a position in an area officially designated as medically underserved (i.e., where there is a shortage of doctors relative to the population). These waivers, which may be offered by a range of state, regional, and national agencies, are usually in rural areas, inner city areas, or unique venues such as Native American reservations. Participating IMGs must commit to a minimum of three years medical practice but do receive salaries and sometimes additional benefits for their service. At the end of that time they may be eligible for Permanent Resident (Green Card) status. There are currently no reliable data on how many or what percentage of IMGs on J-1 visas pursue and obtain these waivers, but it is estimated to be a very high percentage of those inclined and eligible to do so.

IMGs on H-1B visas are generally subject to a six-year limitation of their stay in the United States and must pursue other immigrant options, most commonly that of Permanent Resident based on employer or family-based sponsorship, to remain beyond that time.

Regardless of the route to Permanent Resident status, once it is achieved the IMG is then free to pursue any and all professional options for which he or she can qualify on the basis of training and credentials.

2 Obtaining a Residency Position in the United States

Gerald P. Whelan, MD, Stephen S. Seeling, JD, and Vijay Rajput, MD

Application Process and Requirements — 11

Educational Commission for Foreign Medical Graduates (ECFMG) Certification — 12

United States Medical Licensing Examination (USMLE) — 13

■ *Some Practical Points* — 13

■ *Test Preparation* — 14

■ *ECFMG Standard Certificate* — 14

■ *USMLE Step 3* — 15

■ *Summary of USMLE Steps* — 15

Credential Verification and Transcripts — 15

Obtaining Information about Specific Programs — 16

Sources of Information — 16

■ *FREIDA Online (Fellowship and Residency Electronic Interactive Database Access)* — 17

■ *The Graduate Medical Education Directory (The Green Book)* — 18

■ *Program Web Sites* — 20

Selection of Specialty — 20

■ *Medical or Surgical Specialty* — 20

■ *Type of Institution or Hospital* — 21

■ *Location* — 22

■ *International Medical Graduate (IMG) History* — 22

■ *IMG Performance in the National Resident Matching Program (NRMP) Match* — 23

Summary — 23

Application Process and Requirements

The certification process begins by applying to the Educational Commission for Foreign Medical Graduates (ECFMG) for a USMLE/ECFMG Identification Number. It is critical to record and securely store this number because it will be used throughout the ECFMG certification process and only one number will be issued to any individual applicant. The information provided during the process of obtaining the Identification Number becomes a part of an applicant's permanent ECFMG record. The process of obtaining a USMLE/ECFMG number can be initiated at any time by an international medical graduate (IMG) who is currently enrolled in or is a graduate of a medical school listed in the International Medical Education Directory (IMED, see below), but no examinations can be taken until the basic medical science component of the medical school curriculum has been completed, generally the first two years of a medical school curriculum. Before applying for any examination, applicants must also read the applicable editions (those that pertain to the eligibility period in which they plan to take the exam) of the ECFMG *Information Booklet* and the USMLE *Bulletin of Information*. These publications can be accessed at www.ecfmg.org.

At the time of registration for examinations, IMG students who are still enrolled in medical school must have their good standing as students verified by their medical school, whereas those who are graduates of a medical school must submit a copy of their final medical diploma to ECFMG for verification by that medical school. A completed application will then allow IMGs to register and sit for the necessary United States Medical Licensing Examination (USMLE), which must be passed for ECFMG certification.

ECFMG CERTIFICATION

In order to begin training in a residency or fellowship accredited by the Accreditation Council for Graduate Medical Education (ACGME), IMGs must receive certification by ECFMG, a non-governmental, non-profit organization with organizational members comprising the major professional organizations involved in American medicine, medical education, and licensure .

The best and most reliable source of information regarding ECFMG Certification is, of course, from ECFMG itself. Its Web site (www.ecfmg.org) has news and forms, many of which can be completed and submitted on-line. This book provides a broader overview of the certification process than the ECFMG Web site, but because requirements are detailed and may change, the ECFMG Web site or ECFMG Information Bulletin should always be consulted before taking any actions with respect to certification.

The ECFMG Applicant Information Service (AIS) provides answers to specific questions about ECFMG Certification and related topics; it can be reached by telephone at 215/386-5900 or by e-mail at info@ecfmg.org. Applicants can also subscribe to a free electronic newsletter, *The ECFMG Reporter* (www.ecfmg.org/reporter). It provides useful and timely information related to all aspects of ECFMG Certification.

For ECFMG Certification purposes, an IMG is defined as a physician who received his or her basic medical degree or qualification from a medical school located outside the United States and Canada. To be eligible for ECFMG certification, the physician's medical school and graduation year must be listed in the International Medical Education Directory (IMED) maintained by the Foundation for the Advancement of International

Medical Education and Research (FAIMER) and available on its Web site (www.faimer.org). IMGs must document the completion of all requirements for, and receipt of, the final medical diploma and transcript.

UNITED STATES MEDICAL LICENSING EXAMINATION (USMLE)

To receive ECFMG Certification, IMGs must pass three steps of the USMLE (Box 2-1). These examinations are identical to those required of U.S. medical students. Step 1 and Step 2 CK are computer-based, multiple-choice-question (MCQ) examinations and are offered at test centers operated by the Thomson Prometric Testing Services throughout the United States and around the world. Step 2 CS is a standardized patient (SP) based examination that simulates typical doctor-patient clinical encounters; it is offered in only five cities, all in the United States. More information about these examinations can be found on the USMLE Web site (www.usmle.org). There are separate "Seven Year Rules" that apply to the time within which examinations must be completed successfully to qualify for the ECFMG Standard Certificate or state medical licenses. Because these rules are complex and differ for ECFMG certification and licensure, refer to the ECFMG Bulletin of Information, ECFMG Applicant Information Services at 215/386-5900, or the Federation of State Medical Boards Web site (www.fsmb.org) for current information.

☑ BOX 2-1 **USMLE Steps That Must Be Passed to Receive ECFMG Certification**

■ *Step* 1 (Basic Science)
■ *Step* 2 CK (Clinical Knowledge)
■ *Step* 2 CS (Clinical Skills)

Some Practical Points

IMGs should not attempt the Step 1 or Step 2 CK exams prematurely—that is, before they are optimally prepared to do so. It is important to score as high as possible, because once an examination is passed it may not be repeated for the purpose of trying to achieve a better score. Marginally passing scores can make it very difficult to gain entry into a training program, so it is best for students to take these exams only when they are fully prepared.

Step 2 CS is offered at test centers operated by the Clinical Skills Evaluation Collaboration (CSEC) in, as mentioned previously, only five cities, all in the United States. Therefore IMGs coming from outside the United States for this exam need to be prepared for the expense of travel and accommodation. Those coming from countries for which a travel visa is required must also obtain the appropriate visa, usually a B-1 Visitors visa. Often, IMGs traveling for the Step 2 CS exam will try to coordinate interviews with potential programs (see the Interviewing section in Chapter 3).

Step 2 CS simulates physician-patient clinical encounters using SPs, so it is desirable that the aspiring IMG have similar clinical experience before attempting this examination. Exerience with SPs would also be helpful.

An essential part of the Step 2 CS is the assessment of Spoken English Proficiency (SEP). This is an independent component of the exam, and the IMG must receive a passing score in this component to pass the overall CS exam, regardless of performance on the other components. IMGs whose first language is not English might consider some self-assessment before registering to take CS.

A revised Test of English as a Foreign Language (TOEFL), which includes assessment of spoken English, is readily available in most countries (see www.ets.org for information on both). This test is not expensive and can provide useful information to applicants preparing for the CS examination. Failure to achieve a reasonable score on the TOEFL may suggest that the IMG is not prepared to take the CS exam without some additional spoken English training or practice.

Test Preparation

The National Board of Medical Examiners offers self-assessment services using content similar to that on Step 1 and Step 2 CK on-line via their Web site (www.nbme.org). These examinations are reasonably priced and provide very useful and specific feedback. There are numerous examination preparation books and manuals written specifically for the various USMLE examinations.

There are also a number of test preparation courses offered by commercial firms. The courses for the Step 2 CS may include practice with and feedback from SPs. However, these courses are generally quite expensive and cannot guarantee that the IMG will pass the actual USMLE examination, and none are endorsed or specifically recommended by NBME, ECFMG, or USMLE. The American College of Physicians (ACP) offers a clinical skills practice examination workshop (four stations) with verbal and written feedback at its annual scientific meeting specifically for students preparing for the CS examination. This is at no extra cost to the student beyond meeting registration, which in certain circumstances is free if the student is a member of a regional ACP chapter. More information is available at www.acponline.org.

It is scarcely necessary to remind IMGs that penalties for cheating on the USMLE examinations can be severe (Box 2-2).

☑ **BOX 2-2   A Word of Caution!**

■ Sharing or receiving questions or cases from actual USMLE examinations via the Internet or any written or oral means is *absolutely forbidden*. USMLE staff intensively monitor for this.
■ IMGs found to be participating in this or any other form of "irregular behavior" may have their USMLE transcripts permanently annotated to that effect and may be barred from taking further USMLE examinations for extended periods of time, possibly several years.

ECFMG Standard Certificate

In contrast to prior practice, the examinations listed on Standard Certificates currently being issued by ECFMG are valid indefinitely and have no expiration date or date for revalidation. The ECFMG Certificate is required for entry into any accredited residency or fellowship program and is also required for unrestricted medical licensure for IMGs in all U.S. states and jurisdictions. It must be presented to the program director upon entry into the program, and the program director must verify its authenticity with ECFMG. The ECFMG Standard Certificate is a valuable document that may be required at several points in an IMG's professional career; on return from the program director, the Certificate should be kept in a secure place.

USMLE Step 3

The USMLE Step 3 examination is not required for ECFMG certification; rather, ECFMG Certification is a prerequisite to sit the Step 3 examination. This additional test is required for IMGs entering programs on H-1B visas. It is also required for all IMGs, as well as all USMGs (United States medical graduates), to obtain an unrestricted license to practice medicine anywhere in the United States or its territories. Applicants for Step 3 must be sponsored by a licensing jurisdiction, and eligibility criteria vary among them. Some require no GME while others may require a variable time of GME experience, in some states up to three years, before being eligible to sit the Step 3 examination. Information regarding eligibility can be obtained from the Federation of State Medical Boards (www.fsmb.org).

Step 3 is a computer-based examination composed primarily of MCQs but also includes a number of Clinical Case Simulations (CCSs), which are dynamic, interactive simulations of clinical case diagnosis and management. Because this format is unique to the USMLE examinations, applicants should familiarize themselves with the format by reviewing and using practice materials downloadable from the USMLE Web site (www.usmle.org). Self-assessment materials for Step 3 are also available at www.nbme.org.

Summary of USMLE Steps

- *Step* 1 assesses whether you understand and can apply important concepts of the sciences basic to the practice of medicine, with special emphasis on principles and mechanisms underlying health, disease, and modes of therapy. Step 1 ensures mastery not only of the sciences that provide a foundation for the safe and competent practice of medicine in the present but of the scientific principles required for maintenance of competence through lifelong learning.
- *Step* 2 assesses whether you can apply medical knowledge, skills, and understanding of clinical science essential for the provision of patient care under supervision and emphasizes both health promotion and disease prevention. Step 2 ensures that due attention is devoted to principles of clinical sciences and basic patient-centered skills that provide the foundation for the safe and competent practice of medicine.
- *Step* 3 assesses whether you can apply medical knowledge and understanding of biomedical and clinical science essential for the unsupervised practice of medicine, with emphasis on patient management in ambulatory settings. Step 3 provides a final assessment of physicians assuming independent responsibility for delivering general medical care.

Refer to the USMLE Web site for detailed information regarding the content tested in each examination.

CREDENTIAL VERIFICATION AND TRANSCRIPTS

IMGs must provide proof that they have completed their medical school education. To do so, they must submit a copy of their final medical school diploma to ECFMG who, in turn, will send it directly to the IMG's medical school to verify its authenticity. This process is called *primary source verification*. Finally, an official copy of the IMG's final medical school transcript must be sent to ECFMG by the student's medical school.

When all the required examinations are passed within the specified period of time, the diploma has received primary source verification, and the transcript has been received and all fees paid, ECFMG issues an ECFMG Standard Certificate (see above).

Obtaining Information about Specific Programs

SOURCES OF INFORMATION

There are over 8300 accredited graduate medical education programs, as well as 200 combined residency programs, in the United States. Obtaining accurate, unbiased, and up-to-date information on all these programs would be a truly daunting task were it not for the fact that excellent resources are freely available to IMGs anywhere in the world via the Internet and other sources.

FREIDA Online

Probably the most useful source of information with respect to GME programs for the aspiring resident or fellow is FREIDA Online (Fellowship and Residency Electronic Interactive Database Access). The information on FREIDA is compiled via an annual survey of residency/fellowship programs and is published electronically and maintained by the American Medical Association (AMA) at www.ama-assn.org/go/freida. FREIDA can be accessed by interested users without the need to register or log in; there is no fee. AMA members, including student and resident members, can save searches and print mailing labels. FREIDA's contents are discussed below.

Residency/Fellowship Training Program Search Function

The FREIDA residency/fellowship training program search function allows users to select programs by medical specialty, by location within the United States, and/or by an extensive set of optional criteria (Box 2-3).

☑ **BOX 2-3** **FREIDA Online: Residency/Fellowship Training Program Optional Criteria**

- Participation in National Resident Matching Program (NRMP)
- Participation in Electronic Residency Application Service (ERAS)
- Requirements for prior GME
- Availability of preliminary positions
- Availability of part-time or shared positions
- Start dates other than June or July
- Availability of special training tracks (e.g., primary care, rural, women's health, and hospitalist tracks) and research track/nonaccredited fellowships
- Program setting (e.g., university or community hospital)
- Program size

Search results display information regarding as many or as few programs as meet the user's specifications, including: contact information; general information such as the size and design of the program; information about faculty, typical work schedules, and the program's educational environment; and compensation and benefits information such as salary levels.

Any user can view and download information from FREIDA during a single session, but only AMA members can electronically maintain folders of programs on the Web site for future reference and print mailing labels for programs. Information about becoming an AMA member is available on the Web site.

Training Statistics

The FREIDA training statistics section provides information at the medical specialty level such as the number of programs and length of training, the total number of resident/ fellow positions, and, of particular interest to IMGs, the average percentage of IMGs per program in each particular specialty. It also includes information on faculty, work hours, and work environment and compensation.

When viewing this information it is important to remember that the data reflect averages across the particular medical specialty and that there may be significant variation from one program to another within that medical specialty. Hence, the value of this section for IMGs is primarily to get an understanding of the number of available positions in any given specialty as well as the likelihood, based on past experience, of IMGs obtaining a position in that specialty. These issues are discussed more fully in the section on selecting a specialty.

Graduate Career Plans Statistics

Another FREIDA section reports on the plans of graduating residents, including whether or not they intend to pursue additional training, where they plan to practice, and whether they are pursuing primarily practice or academic careers. There are a number of caveats regarding this information of which the reader should be aware: the information is based on reports from Program Directors; not all graduating residents and fellows have or share their plans; and obviously not all graduates are successful in pursuing their plans.

Perhaps of most interest to IMGs in this section is the percentage of graduates pursuing additional training, because this indirectly reflects the viability and desirability of practicing after a basic residency versus the need to pursue additional training.

ABOUT FREIDA ONLINE

A self-referential section provides information about FREIDA itself and includes an extensive list of frequently asked questions (FAQs), a glossary of terms relating to GME programs, and contact information for FREIDA staff.

The glossary is of particular value and should be read in its entirety before even beginning the process of looking at other program information.

GME RESOURCES AND LINKS

FREIDA contains a section listing resources and links regarding GME. Although the material on medical licensure provides useful links and contact information for the agencies and organizations involved in licensure, much of the general information is more relevant to practicing physicians than to newly arriving IMGs entering residency or fellowship. More specific information is provided in the section of this book on licensure for IMGs.

Probably the most useful resource in this section of FREIDA is the Graduate Medical Education Directory, commonly known as the Green Book. It is described in detail below.

Using FREIDA Effectively

Although FREIDA provides comprehensive information on individual GME programs and some very useful background information regarding specialties and terminology related to GME, the very size and scope of the database can be overwhelming. Therefore, although it is ultimately an exceptionally useful tool in learning about and identifying programs, it is probably not the first tool that an IMG should use in searching for suitable and desirable programs. If the IMG can first make some preliminary decisions regarding the specialty that he or she intends to pursue, the most desirable location(s) of training programs, and the preferred size and type of program, then the search conducted on FREIDA can be considerably more focused and return a more manageable list of potential programs for further exploration.

The Graduate Medical Education Directory (The Green Book)

This directory, commonly referred to as the Green Book, is published annually by the American Medical Association. It is available in hard copy and on CD-ROM but is not available online. It can be purchased by individuals but can frequently be found in the reference section of medical school and university libraries.

Section I contains very useful information on residency application and career planning and links to additional sources. It proposes an annual timeline for preparing for and participating in the residency application process, gives overviews and contact information for ERAS and NRMP, and provides information and links to several useful resources including those listed in Box 2-4.

✔ **BOX 2-4** **Contents of Section I of the Green Book**

■ Choosing a Medical Specialty
■ Transitioning to Residency: What Medical Students Need to Know
■ The Residency Interview: A Guide for Medical Students
■ Find a Residency or Fellowship
■ AMA Alliance of Resident Physicians Spouses and Medical Students Spouses

---

Section I also contains fairly detailed GME information for IMGs. Similar information is included herein in a somewhat more readable format (see section on ECFMG Certification), but specific information regarding ECFMG certification and the J-1 Exchange Visitor Program should always be obtained directly from ECFMG because requirements and regulations are always subject to change.

The final component of Section I provides an overview and contact information for GME-related organizations such as the Accreditation Council for Graduate Medical Education (ACGME), the American Association of Medical Colleges (AAMC), and the Association for Hospital Medical Education (AHME).

Section II provides information on the specialties/subspecialties with residency/fellowship programs accredited by ACGME. Information here is similar to the Training Statistics section in FREIDA but with more detail. For each specialty/subspecialty there is a brief Professional Description of the typical practice for each specialty/subspecialty, a listing of any prerequisites, the duration of training, and, where applicable for specialties, a list of available subspecialties. As noted in the prior reference to the FREIDA Training Statistics, readers should be aware that this information is based on aggregate data across all programs in the specialty/subspecialty; individual programs may vary considerably.

Section III provides program-specific information for each of the 8000+ ACGME-accredited residency and fellowship programs. Programs are listed alphabetically by specialty/subspecialty, then alphabetically by state location. Each listing contains the title of the program and identifies the sponsoring institution(s) (medical school, university, hospital, etc.). It gives the program director's name and address, telephone and fax numbers, and e-mail addresses. It also notes the program length in years and the number of residency or fellowship positions approved/offered each year. The final piece of information is the Program ID number. This number is critical and must be accurately recorded for participants in ERAS and/or the NRMP.

Section V contains information regarding GME Teaching Institutions and explains the relationship between hospitals and medical schools where such exist. This may be of some interest but is generally not critical to the typical IMG's selection of programs for application. It does, however, provide a gauge of the size of each institution, based on the number of programs sponsored or affiliated by a given institution.

There is a separate listing in Appendix A of the Green Book of all combined specialty programs, which provides overview information and data of the combined specialties as well as individual program listings. These programs are not accredited by the ACGME as a single entity but are rather approved by member boards of the American Board of Medical Specialties (ABMS). The information provided here is similar to that found in Sections II and III for specialties/subspecialties. IMG applicants should be aware that combined programs generally tend to be highly competitive and generally select few IMGs.

In Appendix B the 24-member specialty boards of the American Board of Medical Specialties (ABMS) describe the requirements for Board Certification in each of their specialties, including training requirements in ACGME-accredited programs, and they provide information about applying for and taking specialty board examinations. There is a good deal of additional information provided by each specialty board, the nature of which is quite variable. However, applicants would be well advised to review in detail the requirements of all boards of the specialties to which they are applying.

Appendix D contains a useful glossary of GME terms, many of which are included in the Glossary section of this publication.

The final section of relevance to IMG applicants is Appendix F, which provides information on medical licensure. A valid, unrestricted medical license is required for the independent practice of medicine anywhere in the United States, and licenses are issued by each jurisdiction, generally each state. The regulations and requirements vary considerably, and this section contains tables that provide state-by-state information. (Note that, although the information in the Green Book is accurate, the section contained herein on medical licensure is considerably easier to read and more specifically directed to IMG issues.) The most authoritative information on medical licensure, however, is always to be obtained from the Federation of State Medical Boards (www.fsmb.org) or from the individual state medical boards whose contact information is listed in the Green Book.

Other AMA Resources

Besides the Green Book, there are several other valuable AMA resources:

1. AMA International Medical Graduate Section (www.ama-assn.org/go/imgs).
2. AMA GME e-Letter, a free monthly e-mail newsletter for anyone interested in current trends in graduate medical education, physician workforce, new

specialties/subspecialties, and related issues. For the current issue, visit www. ama-assn.org/go/gmenews; to subscribe, go to www.ama-assn.org/go/enews.

Program Web Sites

Most GME programs now have Web sites with a great deal of information about the program, the institution where it is offered, and other information that may be useful to potential applicants. Perhaps the easiest way to obtain Web site addresses is through FREIDA. In using the Residency/Fellowship Training Program Search function, when program information is returned in response to the user's search criteria, included for that program is the URL for its Web site if the program has one and chooses to include that information in FREIDA.

Program Web sites vary, but many contain valuable information, such as rotations, call schedules, faculty profiles, and research publications, that can help the potential applicant obtain a fuller understanding of the program and its features. However, users should be aware that the Web sites are designed and posted by the programs themselves and therefore will portray an image of their own programs as positively as possible.

SELECTION OF SPECIALTY

GME programs in the United States differ greatly from one another. There are many ways that they can be categorized and compared, but perhaps the most obvious are by:

- Medical or surgical specialty
- Program setting (i.e., type of institution or hospital where the program is offered)
- Location

Medical or Surgical Specialty

Beyond the basic decision to become a doctor in the first place, the choice that will most significantly affect a physician's medical career and lifestyle is the choice of the medical or surgical specialty to be pursued and hopefully practiced for the rest of his or her professional life.

In American medicine there is considerable variation in the way that various specialties are perceived, and this leads to some significant differences in how much competition there is to obtain GME positions in different specialties. Some of the appeal of certain specialties may have to do with their potential to ultimately allow those physicians to have very high incomes or very comfortable lifestyles. Some specialties are competitive primarily because they are held in especially high esteem by both the medical community and the public. Often, competition is a function of a relatively limited number of training positions or programs. It is also worth noting that the attractiveness and competitiveness of specialties change over time.

Therefore it certainly makes sense for an IMG considering a program in a given specialty to realistically consider factors like how many positions and programs there are, how much competition there is likely to be (especially from USMGs), and how strong an applicant they are likely to be seen as based on prior academic performance including, but not limited to, USMLE Step 1 and 2 scores and clinical experience.

At the same time, however, entering a specialty program wherein the IMG is very likely to be unhappy or malcontented is likewise inviting failure and disappointment, with a good deal of unhappiness for all involved (including family and spouses) along the way.

An IMG who is profoundly uncomfortable dealing with emotions or personal conflicts is not likely to do well in psychiatry, just as one who has a profound dislike of children will not be a happy pediatrician. So, as with all important choices in life, there must be a realistic balance struck between what is possible and what is likely to be fulfilling and satisfying. Many doctors have found rich, fulfilling professional and personal lives in specialties that were not their first choice; at times, however, there can exist a degree of mismatch for which even income and lifestyle cannot compensate.

It is also worthwhile addressing the strategy that some IMGs espouse, namely, to enter a GME program in a specialty that is not really one in which they are interested but, after "getting a foot in the door," to subsequently transfer to another program in a specialty in which the IMG is genuinely interested. The problem with this strategy is that although it occasionally works, more often it does not work, and the IMG is left in a specialty program wherein he or she is not likely to ever be happy or professionally satisfied. So, generally speaking, it is probably not wise to accept a position in a program in a specialty in which one is likely to be chronically dissatisfied, because in all likelihood that is exactly where one will remain.

Type of Institution or Hospital

GME programs in the United States are offered in a remarkably wide range of hospitals and institutions. One of the search criteria for users of FREIDA (see above) is program setting. The options are university-based program, community-based university-affiliated program, community-based program, military-based program, and Veterans Administration program.

University-Based Program

The majority of experience in a university-based program takes place in a hospital that serves as a primary affiliate of the medical school. These programs are based at major medical education and research institutions, generally part of a university system that also includes disciplines beyond medicine. They tend to be highly competitive and often stress clinical research as part of their program.

Community-Based University-Affiliated Program

The majority of experience takes place in a community hospital that is affiliated with an academic medical center but is not a primary affiliate or is geographically separate from the academic medical center.

Community-Based Program

The majority of experience in a community-based program does not take place in a university academic medical center or a hospital with a medical school affiliation.

Military-Based Program

The majority of experience in a military-based program takes place in Army, Air Force, Navy, and Uniformed Services institutions. These programs are not generally accessible to IMGs.

Veterans Administration Program

A Veterans Administration program is not a category listed in the FREIDA options. Nevertheless, applicants should be aware that a number of programs, although affiliated with academic institutions, offer experience primarily, or to a large extent, at hospitals and outpatient facilities of the Veterans Administration. These facilities offer medical care to qualified veterans of the Armed Forces. Historically, this was primarily an adult male population; now an increasing number of women veterans are eligible for care at a VA facility.

Residency positions that are directly appointed by the VA are not available to non-U.S. citizens regardless of visa status. However, if appointments are made by the affiliated academic institutions, there is no such restriction.

The categorization of programs as listed in FREIDA is based on self reporting by the programs. So, although the foregoing describes a fairly well-delineated hierarchy of programs, they vary as to how neatly they fit into these categories, and it is worthwhile to clarify at the time of the interview, if not before, which of these prototypes best fits any given program. But, again, the general rule holds: The more competitive the program, the more difficult it is for any applicant to gain acceptance. The point is for each applicant to honestly assess his or her individual resume and realistically decide the likelihood of being considered for entry into the various types of programs.

Location

The larger urban centers (New York, Boston, Philadelphia, Chicago, and Los Angeles) within the United States tend to have the largest number of medical and medical education facilities, including the whole spectrum of types of programs noted above. Not surprisingly, these are also the areas where the highest numbers of IMGs find positions. It is worth noting that these are also the areas in which there are the highest numbers of immigrants, so there is often some advantage seen in having physicians of a particular ethnic group caring for patients of the same or similar groups.

For IMGs coming from certain parts of the world and various climates, weather may be a real consideration. Those coming from tropical or subtropical climes might think twice before subjecting themselves (and their families) to a frigid New England winter. On the other hand, those coming with the intention of staying to practice and live in the United States should be aware that residents, both USMGs and IMGs, tend to stay and set up practice in the geographic area in which they train. This is likely a function of contacts that they make with the local medical community while they are residents or fellows but may be less of a factor for IMGs on J-1 Exchange Visitor Visas who obtain waivers to work in underserved areas.

IMGs who are coming to train in the United States and who are bringing a spouse and/or children should also consider the opportunities for employment for their spouse and for child care and schooling for their children, as well as cultural and recreational activities for the entire family. Although acculturation into American society is to be very strongly encouraged, there is also much to be said for having some contact with people from one's native country, and this is a very legitimate factor in deciding where to locate.

IMG History

One final factor worth considering in evaluating the likelihood of acceptance into a given program would be the program's history with respect to IMGs. Review of programs' resident complements will reveal a range of programs from those that rarely if ever accept IMGs to those in which most or even all residents are IMGs. Obviously, a program that has a history of accepting IMGs in the past is more likely to do so in the future. It may be even more informative if it can be determined whether previous graduates from the IMG's own medical school or institution have been accepted in a particular program. Programs that are satisfied with the work of graduates from particular medical schools or institutions are more likely to look favorably on subsequent applicants from those schools.

IMG Performance in the NRMP Match

The National Resident Matching Program (see Chapter 3) reports the number of residency positions offered through the Match each year and also reports the number of positions filled by applicant category. In the 2007 Match, 21,845 PGY-1 positions and 2840 PGY-2 positions or a total of 24,685 positions, were offered, an all-time high and an increase of 600 (2.5%) over the 2006 number. In reporting Match results, NRMP differentiates U.S. IMGs from non-U.S. IMGs. In 2007, 1117 of 2015 (55.4%) active U.S. IMG applicants and 2970 of 5671 (52.4%) active non-U.S. IMG applicants obtained positions through the Match. Although those match rates are somewhat lower than in previous years, the absolute number of both active applicants and successfully matching applicants in both categories was at an all-time high, and the number of IMGs as a percentage of all matched applicants in 2007 (22%) has remained remarkably constant over the past several years.

It should be noted that not all residency positions are filled through the Match. In the 2006 Match, 1231 U.S. IMGs and 3151 non-U.S. IMGs obtained residency positions, but, according to AMA statistics, 6613 IMGs with no prior U.S. GME were on duty in their first year of GME on December 1 of that year.* This suggests that some 2227 IMGs (34%) obtained positions outside of the Match proper. Some may have gotten positions in the post-Match "Scramble", but many others would have accepted positions outside the Match (see Chapter 3).

Summary

The options available for IMGs seeking entry into U.S. GME programs are realistically somewhat more restricted than for U.S. graduates. Decisions should take into account preferred specialty, type of program, and geographical location, but ultimately decisions often come down to the realistic likelihood of gaining entry into a given program. When it comes time to submit a Match list or to choose among a number of offers outside the Match, all of these factors must be considered. The likelihood of three or more years of training in a particular program and living in a particular area of the United States and spending one's entire professional career in a particular kind of practice should engender some serious consideration and, in the case of an IMG with spouse or family, some serious discussion. Although many perceive value in gaining entry into American medicine through any specialty or program, such a perspective must be carefully weighed against the long-term prospects for professional and personal satisfaction for oneself and one's family.

*JAMA. 5 September 2007;298(9):Appendix II, Table 5.

3 Applying to Programs

Gerald P. Whelan, MD, *Anna M. Iacone, Vijay Rajput*, MD, *Emily Hartsough, Anna Headly*, MD, *Patrick C. Alguire*, MD, *and Barbara Porter*, MD

Externships and Observerships   27

Resources for Identifying Externships   28

Guidelines for Starting an Externship or Observership   28

The ACGME Core Competencies   29

- *Patient Care*   29
- *Medical Knowledge*   29
- *Practice-Based Learning and Improvement*   30
- *Interpersonal and Communication Skills*   30
- *Professionalism*   30
- *System-Based Practice*   31

Networking in Health Care Professions   31

How To be Visible without Really Trying   32

Research Prior to Training   32

Advanced Degrees Prior to Residency Training   32

Marketing Yourself   33

Preparing a Curriculum Vitae, Resume, and Personal Statement   33

- *Curriculum Vitae*   33
- *Resume*   35
- *Personal Statement*   36

Dean's Letter   36

Letters of Recommendation (LORs)   38

- *Whom Should You Ask to Write a Letter of Recommendation?*   38
- *Requesting a Letter of Recommendation*   39
- *Fraudulent Letters of Recommendation*   39

Interviewing for Residency Positions   39

- *Preparing for the Interview*   39
- *The Interview*   40
- *Post-Interview Communication*   41

Electronic Residency Application Service (ERAS)   42

■ *Overview*   42

■ ERAS *Support Services at* ECFMG   44

■ ERAS *Application and Match Cycle*   44

■ ERAS *Supporting Documents*   44

NRMP Match   51

■ *Purpose of the Match*   51

■ *Participation*   51

■ *Creating the Rank Order List*   52

■ *How the Match Works*   53

■ *Positions Outside the Match*   55

Externships and Observerships

Vijay Rajput and Emily Hartsough

Externships and observerships are two types of clinical experiences available to all medical students, including international medical graduates (IMGs). IMGs participating in externships gain valuable experience with the U.S. medical education and health care systems and may increase their experience in specific areas of medicine. Externships are offered by most U.S. medical schools to current third- or fourth-year U.S. medical students as well as to international medical students and medical graduates. Applicants for externship are reviewed and selected by the medical school's Student Affairs Office. These externships compare closely to U.S. medical school sub-internships or third-year clerkships. Externship information for each school can most easily be found on its Web site. Visa and travel arrangements must be made by the student before coming (see Chapter 4), and a fee to the medical school may be involved. When an externship is completed it can be documented on the student's transcript.

IMGs in an *externship* program participate in direct patient care activities under supervision of residents and attending physicians. This is by far the best way for IMGs to become familiar with the U.S. health care system, as well as an opportunity to display their medical knowledge and skills. Positive letters of recommendation from faculty with whom they have worked during an externship are extremely valuable in applying to programs. In fact, an increasing number of programs will not even consider IMG applicants without U.S. clinical experience.

Obtaining an externship can be a very competitive process for IMGs. You will be competing with U.S. medical students who are applying to programs where the externships are offered, sometimes called "audition rotations." Networking with colleagues already in U.S. GME programs may be helpful in identifying opportunities and having your application seriously considered. Some ethnic medical societies also help their members to obtain externships, and there are commercial firms offering similar services at a fee.

In contrast to an externship, an *observership* is an experience provided by a hospital or residency program that does not allow any involvement in patient care but does allow the IMG to observe how medicine is practiced in U.S. programs. They will usually also allow access to educational activities in the department or program. Each program has different rules for their observers, and many programs will charge an administrative fee. Because the IMG is not actively involved in patient care, these experiences are considerably less valuable than externships with respect to applying to GME programs but are still better than no experience at all. Letters of reference from faculty where IMGs have observed also generally carry less weight than those from the externships.

Applications for externships or observerships should include a CV and personal statement. Participants must have the appropriate visa or passport, and they will need to make appropriate travel and accommodation arrangements. It is also helpful to bring documentation of immunizations and PPD status.

Externships and observerships generally last for one month; when finished, you should obtain a letter from the program coordinator verifying completion. In the case of an externship, this can be added to the transcript. This is also the time to try to get letters of reference from faculty with whom you have worked.

RESOURCES FOR IDENTIFYING EXTERNSHIPS

IMGs seeking clinical experiences in hospitals associated with U.S. medical schools should become familiar with the Extramural Electives Compendium (EEC), an electronic document published by the AAMC Section for Student Affairs and Programs. Available at www.aamc.org/students/medstudents/electives/start.htm, the EEC contains information for medical students in a searchable database format on the scheduling of elective opportunities at AAMC-member U.S. medical schools. It includes:

- Contact information for elective coordinators on medical school campuses
- Application procedures
- Opportunities for students enrolled in both U.S. medical schools and international medical schools
- Dates for acceptance and assignment of visiting students to elective rotations
- Maximum number of weeks of elective opportunities permitted
- Application, tuition, health, and liability/malpractice insurance fees

IMG users can search for electives by institution or by location within the United States or Canada but, most importantly, can restrict the search to institutions that accept IMGs for electives.

AAMC is also piloting a new program, the Visiting Student Application Service (VSAS), designed to facilitate medical student application for elective clerkships at hospitals associated with U.S. medical schools. IMGs are not eligible to participate at present, but plans are to make this resource available to them in the future. Those interested should periodically visit www.aamc.org/programs/vsas/start.htm for any changes in the program involving IMG participation.

Finally, the above resources only apply to clinical rotations at hospitals associated with U.S. medical schools. There are many other academic medical centers and teaching hospitals that also offer externships and/or observerships, but they must be contacted individually.

GUIDELINES FOR STARTING AN EXTERNSHIP OR OBSERVERSHIP

Schedule an appointment to meet with program staff (externs) or the Volunteer Department (observers), as appropriate, before starting. You may be asked to complete a Volunteer Application and Health Evaluation Form. You should receive information regarding:

- ID badge
- Parking privileges
- Security clearance

Become familiar with the layout of the hospital as soon as possible: medical or surgical floors, ICUs, radiology, laboratories, and cafeteria.

If unsure about first-day procedures, ask to speak with one of the chief residents or program director for a specific team assignment.

Whether as an extern or an observer, clarify exactly what activities you are allowed to perform and in what educational activities you are eligible to participate and find out the schedule of weekly teaching activities from the chief resident or clerkship/program director. Familiarize yourself with the hospital library and the electronic resources available, and identify and remember your team members and their names (residents/interns, attending); note that the team may change periodically (every 2-4 weeks) throughout your rotation.

Obtain pager numbers and other contact information or phone numbers for residents and attending physicians, and update them as the team changes. Conversely, make sure the team has your correct contact information. You should also know the schedules of the team members—that is, when they have ambulatory practice sessions, meetings, personal commitments, or other responsibilities (review this on a daily basis with the residents/interns/attendings as appropriate).

Know where and when the team meets daily. Consistently and reliably arrive on time or early. Be engaged and prepared to contribute at all times, to respond to questions asked on rounds or in teaching conferences, to present brief didactic sessions, or make bedside presentations as requested. Additionally, remember that completing an externship or observership at a program does *not* automatically guarantee you an invitation to interview at that residency program, but it does increase your chances.

THE ACGME CORE COMPETENCIES

The ACGME has identified a set of competencies that all students and residents, regardless of specialty, should master by the end of their training. The purpose of these competencies is to set benchmarks that demonstrate successful educational outcomes. The following description of the competencies allows you to see the "big picture" of medical education at the clinical level, better understand the current educational jargon, develop a deeper understanding of the institutional goals for the educational experience, and anticipate how you may be evaluated. The following description also provides some particular points of emphasis with special relevance to IMGs in externships or observerships.

Patient Care

Learners must be able to provide care that is compassionate, appropriate, and effective for the treatment of health problems and the promotion of health.

■ Gather essential and accurate information about patients.
■ Concisely and accurately record information in the chart (provided this is an approved activity).
■ Efficiently and effectively carry out management plans.
■ Attend to the emotional, as well as physical, needs of your patients.

Medical Knowledge

Learners must demonstrate knowledge about established and evolving biomedical, clinical, and cognate (e.g., epidemiological and social-behavioral) sciences and the application of knowledge to patient care.

■ Attend teaching conferences and contribute as appropriate.
■ Contribute to all clinical discussions as appropriate: ask questions, offer management plans, present the results of literature searches, etc.
■ Offer to present brief (5 minutes) didactic sessions to the team based on focused literature searches.

Practice-Based Learning and Improvement

Learners must be able to investigate and evaluate their patient care practices, appraise and assimilate scientific evidence, and improve their patient care practices.

- On rounds or in clinic, make notes of all questions that arise in patient discussions and add to it questions that occur to you.
- Spend some time each day in the library or online finding the answers to these questions and additional information about patient diagnoses, test results, and treatments.
- When appropriate, make copies of pertinent articles for your personal files and/or to share with team members.
- Volunteer information that you have learned from these studies in appropriate settings with the clinical team.

Interpersonal and Communication Skills

Learners must be able to demonstrate interpersonal and communication skills that result in effective information exchange and teaming with patients, their families, and professional associates.

- Speak up! Team members and attending can only know your capabilities if they are voiced or demonstrated. They cannot read minds!
- Contribute to all conversations. Remain engaged and enthusiastic.
- Speak as clearly and as succinctly as possible.
- Request clarification when necessary, whether related to patient care or hospital procedures.
- Ask for clarification if you are finding the English language to be difficult. This is how one learns, and the occasional misunderstanding of select words or terms will not affect your evaluation. Also, some misunderstandings may not be related to the language itself but to acronyms or terminology specific to the U.S. health care system and associated slang. This is a learning experience!
- When appropriate, let a sense of humor shine through.
- Relax and enjoy the experience!

Professionalism

Learners must demonstrate a commitment to carrying out professional responsibilities, adhering to ethical principles, and being sensitive to a diverse patient population.

- Remember that local medical students will most likely receive the highest priority in all clinical and teaching activities. Nevertheless, be engaged and prepared to contribute at all times.
- Dress neatly and appropriately.
- Tardiness or absences from assigned clinical duties and teaching activities should not occur or be kept to a minimum. If an unavoidable absence/tardiness is anticipated, discuss it with the team/attending as soon as possible.
- Be polite to everyone: patients, families, hospital staff, nurses, residents, and attending.

■ Do *not lie*, or even stretch the truth. If you do not know the answer to a question, *do not make it up*. Have the humility and the honesty — *at all times* — to say "I don't know . . . but I will do my best to find out the answer for you."

■ Meet with the senior resident and attending at the beginning (and with each change in team member) to clarify your role, responsibilities, and expectations. Seek feedback periodically throughout by focusing on the components of the externship or observership evaluation. Though difficult at times, seeking feedback proactively demonstrates maturity and professionalism.

System-Based Practice

Learners must demonstrate an awareness of, and responsiveness to, the larger context of health care and the ability to effectively call on system resources to provide care that is of optimal value.

■ Understand health care delivery at the "micro" and "macro" level. The "micro" level is health care delivery in the hospital and in offices dealing with social work, nursing home and rehabilitation, discharges, utilization review, etc. The "macro" level is health care at the community or global level and involves the application of insurance issues (private and public such as Medicare, Medicaid).

■ Pay attention to discussions about how the components of the health care system can best be used to meet a patient's particular needs. The U.S. health care system is a complicated one. Don't expect to learn it in any great detail right away.

■ Network with health care professional friends and acquaintances. Networking in every profession and business is useful. IMGs may not have many contacts in the United States, but staying in contact with residents who are graduates of your medical school and who are now in U.S. GME programs is very important for developing a residency network. ECFMG has developed a Web-based IMG Advisors Network (IAN) (www.ecfmg.org/acculturation) that can help IMGs who qualify to contact IMGs already in programs for logistical information pertaining to a particular area of the United States.

NETWORKING IN HEALTH CARE PROFESSIONS

Networking is the process of building alliances with other health care professionals. Its purpose is to identify individuals who can help further your career either by their direct actions on your behalf or by contacting others who are capable of making decisions helpful to your needs. IMGs may not have many contacts in the United States, but staying in contact with residents who are graduates of your medical school that are now in U.S. GME programs is very important for developing your residency network. To assist you in this task, ECGMG has developed a Web-based IMG Advisors Network (IAN) (www.ecfmg.org/acculturation) that can help IMGs who qualify to contact IMGs already in programs for logistical information pertaining to a particular area of the United States.

Networking with other residents, students, fellows and academic physicians is essential for finding new observerships, research positions, residency, and future career opportunities. Build a network of friends that will be vigilant for any new opportunities. Increase visibility by attending social events, volunteer meetings, or medical gatherings to meet new contacts from this country.

Other key points related to building a professional network include:

- Offering helpful information to network friends or new physicians in exchange for information and contacts can be very useful. Find people who seem to know everyone, and use e-mails and telephone numbers appropriately to network among new contacts.
- Effective networking with IMG residents in desired programs is more effective than e-mail or letters to those programs. Networking with the right people in residency and particular fields of interest can help reveal hidden opportunities and can set you apart from your other colleagues.
- It is essential to always introduce yourself politely to a target contact like a program director or a key faculty member.
- Focusing on the goal of achieving residency is of absolute importance! Use network friends to find suitable residency programs. Gather all information on these programs and their program directors and faculty. Find out who has the hiring power; many times it is the program directors and senior faculty in the program.
- Engineering a networking introduction and building word-of-mouth exchanges will be very helpful to you. Be able to describe your achievements in one paragraph in addition to the more complete information in your CV and personal statement.
- Being cheerful, confident, and straightforward in all person-to-person communications, and mentioning common interests when possible, will make you stand out from other candidates. It is also extremely important to know when to stop talking. Before picking up the phone to talk to anyone in a program, write down opening lines. This is essential if you are not comfortable with language skills.

HOW TO BE VISIBLE WITHOUT REALLY TRYING

There are several ways in which to draw attention to yourself without being "pushy" or "show-offy". Some suggestions are to:

- Ask appropriate questions at conferences and meetings.
- Discuss a book or new article in a journal with faculty.
- Wear bright ties.
- Make people laugh.
- Have and express opinions.
- Use e-mails and the Internet to communicate interest.

RESEARCH PRIOR TO TRAINING

For information on research prior to training, see Chapter 8.

ADVANCED DEGREES PRIOR TO RESIDENCY TRAINING

Over the past decade medicine has undergone major transformations. Many American-trained medical students are receiving additional advanced professional degrees while completing medical school or after medical school training. Advanced degrees (e.g., PhD, MBA, JD) are popular in enhancing professional development. The most common reason for this is to have a career in clinical medicine as well as in clinical science, research, business, or the medicolegal profession.

Recently many international medical graduates have pursued a research career prior to residency training for many reasons. Sometimes it is easier to start a career in a research laboratory and get an employment visa as a research fellow. It also provides time to pass required examinations. The major downside to getting a PhD is the amount of time it takes to obtain it. This leads to a prolonged hiatus from clinical experience. Many program directors see this as a major obstacle in adjusting to the U.S. clinical system's complex clinical environment.

The other common path chosen by many International medical graduates is to get an MPH degree from a university in the United States. These are mainly one-year programs with basic credits in epidemiological research and some field experience. This has been a common stepping stone to getting into residency. The international medical graduate on a student visa has one-year optional training to complete this experience. This is also called the F-1 *Optional Practical Training* (OPT) *visa*, valuable for gaining experience in the field in which you trained.

Another dual degree that has become attractive to U.S. students is MD/MBA. The *business* of medicine (e.g., governmental regulation, insurance and reimbursement issues) intrigues many students. There are more than fifty medical schools that offer the dual MD/MBA degree. Physicians find new career opportunities in health care management, administration, government relations, and the pharmaceutical and biotech industries. These professional degrees are one- to two-year courses depending on whether they are part-time or full-time courses. IMGs may also wish to learn more about the degrees for master of health administration (MHA) or master of business administration (MBA), which is more general for any type of business, including health care.

Entry into all these professional degree programs requires taking the Graduate Management Admission Test (GMAT) (www.mba.com/mba) or the Graduate Record Examination (GRE) and the Test of English as a Foreign Language (TOEFL) examination (www.ets.org).

Marketing Yourself

PREPARING A CURRICULUM VITAE, RESUME, AND PERSONAL STATEMENT

Anna Headly and Patrick C. Alguire

Curriculum Vitae

You will need to have an up-to-date curriculum vitae (CV) to apply for any training or employment in the U.S. A CV is a detailed summary of your education, experience, research, and accomplishments. A CV includes much more information than a resume, which is typically only a page long and does not describe your research, publications, or presentations. There are no page limits for a CV.

Your CV may be the first thing a prospective program looks at, so you should make sure it appears perfect, with no spelling, punctuation, or grammatical errors. Your CV should be in a standard typeface (e.g., Times Roman or Arial), no smaller than 10 points, and no larger than 12 points. It should have margins of about one inch on all sides. It is helpful to include your last name and page number on each page of your CV after the first page.

A comprehensive sample CV outline is presented in Box 3-1. The following items bear particular attention:

- Full name (given name first, family name last)
- Mailing address, phone number, and e-mail address
- Citizenship (and visa status, if applicable)

☑ **BOX 3-1 Sample Curriculum Vitae Outline**

Personal Information
- Full name
- Citizenship
- Home address, telephone number, e-mail address
- Professional address, telephone number, e-mail address
- Present academic rank and position (if applicable)
    Example: Instructor of Medicine, Medical School
    Example: Consultant, Department of Internal Medicine, Division of Gastroenterology, Medical School

Education
- Name of institution, degree(s), and date(s)
- College/University
- Medical school
- Residency
- Fellowship
- Other

ECFMG Certification
- Certificate number

Board Certification (if applicable)*
- List month and year of successful completion

Medical Licensure (if applicable)
- Indicate state and license number only

Honors and Awards
- *Example*: Resident Teacher of the Year award, undergraduate honors, Alpha Omega Alpha
- List chronologically, beginning with earliest appointment

Military Service (if applicable)
- List branch of service, rank, place, and dates

Academic Appointments and Positions
- *Example*: Academic research, clinical appointments
- List chronologically, beginning with earliest appointment

Teaching
- List dates and names of courses taught, time spent as leader of rounds, seminars presented, student advisor roles filled, etc.
- Medical school
- Graduate school
- Continuing education
- Other institutions (prior to current position)

Journals
- List membership on editorial boards, position as scientific reviewer for medical journals, etc.
- List chronologically, beginning with earliest appointment

Institutional, Departmental and Divisional Administrative Responsibilities, Committee Memberships, and Other Activities
- List all, including years active
- List chronologically, beginning with earliest appointment
- If still active, list date as follows: 2008–

Professional and Society Memberships
- List dates, offices held, and committee responsibilities
- List chronologically, beginning with earliest appointment

Invited Visiting Professorships
- List dates, place, and professorship title
- List chronologically, beginning with earliest appointment

Presentations at National Meetings
- List dates, meeting names, places, and topics
- List chronologically, beginning with earliest presentation

Presentations at International Meetings
- List dates, meeting names, places, and topics
- List chronologically, beginning with earliest presentation

Intramural Presentations
- Presentations at the physician's hospital or institutions; presentations, Mortality and Morbidity Conferences, or Journal Club meeting at Grand Rounds, or formal presentations to medical students
- List chronologically, beginning with earliest presentation

Research Grants
- Grant number and title, time period
- List chronologically, beginning with earliest award

Civic Activities
- List both medically and non-medically related activities

Publications: Journals
- *Published articles*: List chronologically, beginning with earliest publication
- Use "In Press" for those articles accepted but not printed
- Use "Submitted" for those submitted but not yet accepted or rejected
- Use "In Preparation" for those written but not submitted

Publications: Abstracts, Editorials, Book Chapters
- After the title, identify in parentheses whether the work is an abstract, an editorial, or a book chapter; put all abstracts in a separate grouping
- List chronologically, beginning with earliest publication

The following should not appear on your CV:
- Date of birth
- Sex
- Family information
- Social Security or passport numbers
- Education or awards prior to college unless especially noteworthy (e.g., national competitions)
- *Anything* that you would not be willing to discuss in an interview

---

*Do not list headings that do not apply to you. For example, if you do not have Board Certification, do not put down that heading.

- *Education*: In the United States, students typically attend a college or university for four years, then attend medical school for four years. These eight years are separated on a CV as, respectively, "Undergraduate Education" and "Graduate Education." In other parts of the world, it is common for medical education and college to be combined. If you graduated from a combined program, this should be listed under the heading "Education." It is important to note whether you graduated with special honors or distinction; you may also note your class rank.
- *Postgraduate Education*: If you have already completed an internship, residency, or fellowship, these experiences are listed under the heading "Postgraduate Education."
- *Certification*: List important examinations (USMLE Step Examinations, board certifications) and licensures here. If you scored very well on your examinations (at least higher than the mean score), list your scores as well.
- *Work Experience*: List any paid jobs you have held since you graduated from high school. These should be listed in chronological order.
- *Volunteer Experience*: List any unpaid positions you have held, especially those that involve community service. These should also be in chronological order.
- *Research Experience*: List any work in research, whether paid or unpaid. This is not where you list publications or presentations, but rather work you performed on a study or in a laboratory. Keep your description to about two sentences.
- *Honors and Awards*: This section can include anything that you have been awarded based on merit, including scholarships, prizes, memberships in honor societies, etc.
- *Publications/Bibliography*: A CV for application to a residency or fellowship program can list all publications, abstracts, and presentations under one general title. A CV for a job after residency or fellowship should separate publications into "Peer-Reviewed Publications" (i.e., papers published in journals that send their articles out for review) and "Other Publications." There are a few different styles for citing publications; the important thing is to be consistent.
- *Membership in Professional Societies*: If you belong to any medical societies, list them here.
- *Extracurricular Activities* are interests and accomplishments outside of medicine. If you have a special passion or hobby—juggling, raising pigeons, skydiving, martial arts, painting, playing an instrument, etc.—indicate it here. List at least a couple of entries so that you appear well-rounded, but avoid anything too general (e.g., reading) or that makes you appear lazy (e.g., watching TV).
- *Languages*: List languages besides English, especially languages that may be helpful for your career, such as Spanish, French, Arabic, Vietnamese, and Cantonese. In general, you should list any language in which you can carry on a conversation; you need not be perfectly fluent. If you have a very rudimentary knowledge of a useful language such as Spanish, you can say "elementary Spanish" or "some Spanish." It is not useful to list multiple dialects of a language that is spoken only in your home country.

Resume

A resume is shorter than a CV, usually no more than 1 or 2 pages. A resume presents your education and accomplishments strongly, but briefly, and can be reviewed by the employer quickly. Box 3-2 gives an outline of a good resume.

☑ **BOX 3-2** **Sample Outline of a Resume**

At the Top of the Page
▪ Name
▪ Home address
▪ Home phone number
▪ Professional phone number (when appropriate)

Education
▪ List chronologically backward, from most recent schooling to college undergraduate

Work Experience
▪ Include postgraduate training from most recent position to first position

Special Skills
▪ List special attributes such as foreign languages, computer skills, and procedural skills

Honors and Awards
▪ List, from most recent to earliest, professional or academic awards, scholarships

Extracurricular Activities
▪ Sports, hobbies, involvement in non-medical organizations

Personal Statement

The personal statement (PS) is a component of the application process that is often overlooked by international medical graduates, yet it is one of the most important items in an application for positions in the United States. A personal statement is a document that addresses, in your own voice, why you are applying for the position in question. A poorly written (or absent) personal statement can cause your application to be rejected out of hand. For a program director, a personal statement is a way to find out, first of all, whether you can write reasonably well in English (or at least that you are aware enough of your shortcomings in this area to have someone edit your statement). Next, the personal statement gives some insight into what kind of person and physician you are or wish to become. It should not be a repetition of your CV or of all your accomplishments.

A typical personal statement focuses on a critical point in your journey toward deciding on the position for which you are applying, whether it was a personal event (such as personal or family illness) or an encounter with a special patient. If there is something in your application that might make a program director worried about your suitability as a candidate, such as time off during your education, any failures on any examinations, or any administrative actions taken against you, you should probably address that. If you overcame a significant barrier to obtain your education (poverty, political repression in your home country, etc.), that may be a good thing to write about. If you have a noteworthy achievement, you may also want to describe it more fully here than you could in your CV. Program directors often like to read about what kind of career you currently envision (academic, clinical, international, etc.), but be careful not to sound unrealistic in your goals. In a personal statement, you should avoid sounding as if you are bragging, but you should also not be self-deprecatory. You should aim for one full page, with three or four paragraphs. Once you have written your statement, have it proofread by someone who is a native English speaker. Box 3-3 lists items that do *not* belong in a personal statement.

DEAN'S LETTER

Barbara Porter

Unless there are extenuating circumstances that make it impossible to obtain one, your ERAS application should include a letter from your medical school that summarizes your

---

☑ **BOX 3-3 What to Leave Out of a Personal Statement**

- Anything not written by you personally—never copy any part of any one else's personal statement (Note: There are numerous web sites that present examples of personal statements. They can be useful as guidance but NEVER copy and paste any language from these examples.)
- Any discussion of religion
- Any discussion of US politics
- Any discussion of how much money you hope to make in the future
- Swear words
- Exclamation points
- Negative comments about anything or anyone
- Spelling or grammatical mistakes

---

performance during medical school (see section on ERAS Supporting Documents below). In 2002, the AAMC published guidelines for the preparation of this letter and changed the name of this document from a "Dean's Letter" to a "Medical Student Performance Evaluation" (MSPE). This name change reflects the intended purpose of this document; that is, the document is not a letter of recommendation but a letter evaluating a student's performance in relation to his or her peers.

The MSPE should contain six sections: identifying information, unique characteristics, academic history, academic progress, summary, and appendices. When this format is followed, the document is able to describe the student, highlighting what is unique about the student and their path before and through medical school, including honors bestowed during medical school. The student's performance during the clinical years is emphasized, and narrative comments from each clerkship director describing the student's work are included. The student's performance is summarized in relation to the performance of his or her peers. The AAMC recommends including specific information in each section (Box 3-4).

☑ **BOX 3-4 Association of American Medical Colleges (AAMC) Recommendations for Completing the Medical Student Performance Evaluation (MSPE)**

- The *Identifying Information* section includes your legal name and the name and location of your medical school.
- The *Unique Characteristics* section provides an opportunity to describe what distinguishes you from your peers. Typically this section is a short biography that describes prior education and areas of academic and extra-curricular interest. It also allows for an explanation of any special circumstances, particularly hardships, which may have influenced your matriculation through medical school.
- The *Academic History* section includes expected graduation date and also documents and explains atypical circumstances related to medical school (e.g., enrollment in a dual-degree program, leaves of absence, the need for and completion of remedial work).
- The *Academic Progress* section summarizes your academic performance. Summarize your overall (not course-specific) performance during the pre-clinical years in one or two sentences; describe your performance during the clinical years in a more-detailed, course-specific format. In most U.S. medical schools, a student's performance during a clerkship is documented by a letter grade and by summative comments from the clerkship director. These narrative comments are to be included in this section.
- The *Summary* section is a closing paragraph that summarizes your performance in relation to that of your peers. If your medical school uses a class-ranking system, provide your rank here. If it uses letter grades, provide them along with any descriptive terms such as "outstanding", "excellent", "very good", or "good".
- The AAMC recommends submitting *Appendices* that provide a graphical representation of your performance in relation to that of your peers and that give further information about your medical school.

The AAMC has published A *Guide to the Preparation of the Medical Student Performance Evaluation* (also available at www.aamc.org/students/eras/resources/downloads/mspeguide.pdf). It provides a suggested template for your Dean's office when preparing an MSPE.

A student may have had extenuating or unusual circumstances leading to a prolonged matriculation through medical school (e.g., leave of absence, repeated coursework). Multiple sections of the MSPE allow for an explanation of these circumstances, and the academic history section specifically addresses extensions, failures, and any adverse actions imposed on the student.

While the MSPE usually documents the grades and comments a student receives during the clinical years, it is different from the transcript. The MSPE often only summarizes the preclinical performance; it provides narrative evaluations and summarizes a student's performance in relation to his or her peers. An official transcript (a report of the grade obtained in every course and clerkship completed by the student, including courses audited or withdrawn, and grades of failure or incomplete) is required in the ERAS application. (If a transcript is not available, see section on ERAS Supporting Documents below.) Often the MSPE only summarizes the preclinical performance, so the specific data on the transcript may still be important to the residency program.

Most U.S. medical schools grade their students on a 4-point scale (Honors, High Pass, Pass, Fail) or a 5-point letter or number scale (A, B, C, D, F or 1, 2, 3, 4, 5). A grade of Honors or "A" typically represents performance in the top 90th or 95th percentile of a class. Some schools grade on a Pass/Fail basis only, whereas others combine scales (e.g., electives courses are graded Pass/Fail and required courses are on a 4- or 5-point scale). Additionally, during the clinical years, comments from supervising physicians are collected by clerkship directors and are included as a descriptive evaluation with the grade. The evaluation scheme used by the school is typically included in the appendices to the MSPE.

LETTERS OF RECOMMENDATION (LORs)

Barbara Porter

An important part of the application for residency is the letter of recommendation. These letters are used by residency programs to assess an applicant's non-cognitive qualities, including attitudes and motivations, and to help stratify an applicant's performance in relation to his or her peers. Most residency programs in the United States require at least three LORs to supplement your application to residency. At least two of the letters should be from physicians who have observed your clinical work. A few programs want one of your letters to be a "Chairman's Letter" (i.e., a letter from the chairman of your chosen specialty at your school) or a "Departmental Letter" (i.e., a letter written by a member of the department of your chosen specialty at your school) that summarizes your performance during clerkships and electives in that department. Be sure to check the guidelines of each program to which you are applying. MyERAS (see below) allows you to send four letters to a residency program at one time.

Whom Should You Ask to Write a Letter of Recommendation?

Because you want the letter to portray you accurately and favorably, the LOR should come from someone who knows you well, thinks well of you, and works in your chosen specialty.

If you must choose between someone from a different specialty who knows you well and someone in your chosen specialty who does not know you, it is wise to choose the person who knows you better. Consider asking an attending physician with whom you have spent a sufficient amount of time and who can comment specifically on your clinical skills, your relationships with patients, and your work ethic. In general, the more senior the letter writer, the better; but, again, not if the more senior letter writer does not know you or does not think well of you! You should not, however, ask a resident to write an LOR on your behalf. If you feel that a resident can offer useful insights, you can suggest that one of your letter writers consult with him or her. A letter from a U.S. faculty member may seem more valuable than a letter from a physician from your country, but only if the letter writer demonstrates that he or she has observed your clinical skills and work ethic. Again, the most valuable LOR comes from the physician who knows you best.

Because of the appearance of bias and lack of objectivity, it is inappropriate to have a relative or family member (even if you do not share a name) write you an LOR. If your letter writer shares your surname but is not related to you, ask that he or she make a note of that to avoid the appearance of impropriety. Finally, a letter from a research mentor can be valuable, but only if you have two other letters that vouch for your clinical skills.

Requesting a Letter of Recommendation

When you approach a potential letter writer, ask if he or she can write a "strong" LOR for you. Pay attention to the response you get—if there is hesitation or if the person feels that a "strong" LOR cannot be written because he or she does not know you well enough, ask someone else. Be specific about what you would like the writer to comment on. If the person has not written many LORs for U.S. residency, say that you would like the letter to comment on your clinical skills, your work ethic, and your relationships with patients and colleagues. You can further help the letter writer by setting up a short meeting where you share your CV and personal statement and discuss your time working together and anything you may have done well at that time.

When you request an LOR, allow adequate time for its composition and be considerate of the fact that most letter writers will have several other LORs to write. Four to six weeks before a deadline is usually adequate. Be clear with the writer about when the letter is due and provide him or her with any supporting documents, including the downloadable ERAS coversheet and instructions if you are applying through ERAS (see section on ERAS Supporting Documents below). If at all possible, tell the letter writer that you waive your rights to see the LOR and have the writer submit it directly to ERAS, noting that you have waived this right. In general, readers of LORs have more confidence in the honesty of their contents if the subject has waived the right to see them beforehand.

Fraudulent Letters of Recommendation

An LOR that contains fraudulent information can put a swift and permanent end to any hope of obtaining a position in any U.S. residency program (see section on ERAS Supporting Documents below).

INTERVIEWING FOR RESIDENCY POSITIONS

Anna Headly

Preparing for the Interview

All residency programs require applicants to come for an interview. Interviews take place from November through January and usually take a half to a full day. Before your interview, learn as much as you can about the program. Most programs have informational Web pages. It is especially helpful to learn about what a program considers its strengths, because these are good topics of conversation during your interview. You should also learn something about the program leaders, even though you may not get a chance to speak with any of them on the day you are interviewed. Make sure that whenever you interact with *anyone* from a program—before, during, and after the interview—you must be polite and friendly. Applicants are sometimes rejected because they were rude to a secretary, coordinator, or resident, even if they impressed the program leaders.

There may be an informal dinner with residents the night before the interview day. It is not critical to attend these dinners, but they can help you learn more about whether a particular program will be a good fit for you, and they are an opportunity for you to show the residents that you are genuinely interested in the program. If you do attend the dinner, remember that it is not appropriate to bring anyone with you. Dress for the dinner is less formal than for the interview itself but should be modest, not flashy. At dinner, remember that the way you conduct yourself is being noticed. Shake hands and introduce yourself to the hosts; do not have more than one alcoholic drink; mind your table manners; ask polite questions; and thank the hosts at the end of the evening.

The Interview

Dress conservatively. This means dark suits (black, brown, grey, or navy are safe choices) for both men and women. Women may wear pant suits or skirt suits, but skirts should not be too short (knee length or slightly below the knee is appropriate). A man should always wear a plain shirt (cream, white, and light blue are safe choices) and a tie. Shoes should be black (for black or grey suits) or brown (for brown or blue suits). For men, plain lace-up shoes are best; for women, heels should not be higher than two inches. Women should avoid low-cut tops. Whether you are a man or a woman, make sure you are freshly showered and wearing antiperspirant, but do not use any perfume or cologne. It is also best not to wear any large or flashy jewelry. If you have any requirements for dress because of your religion (e.g., a turban, a yarmulke, or a long skirt), simply make sure that the rest of your attire is as unremarkable as possible. Avoid eating garlic or onions the day before your interview; carry mints if you have any concern about your breath. Never chew gum during the interview day.

Make sure that you arrive to the interview in plenty of time (most will start early in the morning), and try to be well-rested. The day usually consists of presentations by various people in charge (chief residents, program directors), one or two formal one-on-one interviews with faculty members or chief residents, and a tour of the facilities. Sometimes you will have a lot of spare time during the day, but often the schedule is tight: do not plan on being able to make phone calls, for instance. If you have strict dietary requirements, you may not be able to eat all of the food provided; eat well before you arrive and just eat and drink whatever you can during the day, without any comment.

During the actual interviews, you should shake hands with the interviewer before sitting down. Do not pull your chair up close to the interviewer; leave it wherever you find it. Remember to smile while you are talking and listening. If you have difficulty with spoken English, do what you can to minimize the difficulty; speak slowly and carefully, and think before you speak. If you do not understand a question, ask the interviewer to rephrase it.

There are a number of questions for which you should be prepared:

■ *Questions about your CV or personal statement.* If you don't want to talk about something, it should not be written on your CV or personal statement.

- *Questions about your prior training and whether you are prepared to work in the U.S. medical system.* If you have no U.S. experience, you should familiarize yourself with some of the differences between the system you trained in and the U.S. system.
- *Questions about what you perceive to be your weaknesses or about tough situations you wish you had handled differently.* Such questions are not an invitation to brag (answers like "I have no weaknesses" or "I am a perfectionist" do not go over well), but neither are they meant to make you insult yourself. Think honestly about this topic, and try to give an answer that sounds straightforward but that will not frighten the interviewer. For example, you might talk about how you are learning to overcome shyness (or learning not to interrupt others). Weaknesses that would raise a red flag with interviewers include things like dishonesty, laziness, and a bad temper.
- *Questions about any weakness in your application.* If you have a bad grade on your transcript or a poor test score, be prepared to talk about what happened. Take full responsibility for any failures; blaming others is never attractive. Be specific about what you did to fix the problem so that it will not happen again.
- *Questions about where you see yourself after residency or in ten years.* Be honest and realistic in your answers to these questions; trying to guess what the interviewer wants to hear usually backfires. If your plans include, for example, a very competitive subspecialty, make sure you can discuss what you need to do to achieve your goals. If you are undecided, say so: such frankness is usually refreshing for interviewers to hear.

You will be asked many times during the interview day about what questions you have. You never want to answer, "I don't have any" or "They've all been answered." However, you should also avoid asking any questions that may reflect negatively on your motivations. This is not the time to ask about call schedules, salary, or workload. You do need to confirm which visa options are acceptable or preferred by the program because this may influence your ranking decisions, but the subject need not be raised with every interviewer. The program director or coordinator should be able to provide this information. You should also avoid negative questions like "Is your program in financial trouble?" or "Why have so many people quit this residency?" Do not ask questions that have already been answered in the presentations; it will appear as if you did not pay attention. It is also not polite to ask questions about your chances of being chosen by the program. If you were invited for an interview, you can assume that you have a good chance of being ranked unless you make a terrible impression at your interview; your exact ranking is not something any interviewer will be able tell you. Questions about the future of the program are appropriate, especially about what changes are expected. Questions about what graduates do after residency are fine. And, whenever you can't think of a question, "Tell me what you like about your job" works in almost every situation.

Post-Interview Communication

After your interview, it is a good idea to send a thank-you note (written or e-mail) to the program director and perhaps to the faculty member who interviewed you. However, you must make sure that your English is impeccable; you do not want to give anyone any concern that you would have trouble writing in a patient's chart. You should also avoid being too generic in your note; mention something specific about the interview day. Use standard business English salutations. For instance, close with "Sincerely," not "Your humble servant" or "Love"! Never say that a program is your first choice unless that is true. (It is fine to say that you plan to rank a program "highly".) If you are looking for an out-of-match spot, you may say this in your note, but only if you are willing to immediately accept an out-of-match spot with that program. Avoid sounding as if you were desperate to match at a program. Do not send more than one thank-you note to any one person, and do not send notes to anyone you did not talk with.

You may want to go back for a "second look" at a program. In general, this will not help your chances of ranking well, but it can help you in your rank list decisions. "Second looks" involve a fair amount of extra work for everyone involved, so request them with caution.

ELECTRONIC RESIDENCY APPLICATION SERVICE (ERAS)

The process of applying to U.S. GME programs is multifaceted:

- You must be aware of program timeframes and deadlines.
- You must understand the on-line registration and requirements from the various medical organizations involved.
- You must submit and assign various document types to support your ERAS application.
- You must understand the selection criteria and recruitment process set by each program.

Applying to U.S. GME programs is a daunting task, but fortunately a resource exists that significantly streamlines and facilitates this part of the application process: the Electronic Residency Application Service (ERAS).

Overview

ERAS was originally developed by the AAMC in the 1990s to allow all medical students and graduates to apply electronically to training programs by using the Internet. For IMGs participating in ERAS, the primary point of contact is ERAS Support Services at ECFMG.

As part of the residency application process, ERAS Support Services acts as the designated Dean's office for all international medical students and graduates. It allows registered IMG applicants to submit the necessary documents in a timely and secure manner and for the documents to be accessible to the GME programs indicated by the applicant. In other words, ERAS Support Services scans and transmits letters of recommendation (LORs), Medical Student Performance Evaluations (MSPEs), medical school transcripts, USMLE transcripts, and other supporting credentials from the applicant to program directors using the Internet. ERAS consists of:

- MyERAS (the Web site where applicants complete their application)
- Dean's Office Workstation (DWS)
- Program Director's Workstation (PDWS)
- ERAS PostOffice

IMGs are given access to the MyERAS site by first requesting a Token through ECFMG's On-line Applicant Status and Information System (OASIS). The Token is a unique identification number required for MyERAS registration and requires payment of a Token fee as posted.

Important Note: The Token is specific to each individual requestor. IMGs should *not* use any Token identification number other than that issued to them specifically. Using someone else's Token identification number has been the cause of delays and transmission discrepancies to the IMG's applied-to programs.

The AAMC's "MyERAS" site is the entry point to the entire ERAS application process. This site is where applicants, once registered, can perform the following functions:

- Create a Profile (including name, contact information, citizenship status, visa type, USMLE number, NRMP participation, ECFMG certification status, etc.)
- Complete and certify the on-line application (Common Application Form, or CAF)
- Create an on-line Personal Statement
- Select and apply to residency training programs after researching programs of interest
- Create and manage the ERAS application and document assignments for all applied-to programs
- Track the status of the ERAS application via the Applicant Document Tracking System (ADTS)

ERAS Support Services at ECFMG highly urges all IMGs to access the ADTS. The ADTS system provides a listing of all their applied-to programs, the date and time documents were made available to the ERAS PostOffice, and the date and time the programs retrieved documents for evaluation.

The ADTS provides real-time information that is 100% accurate. The cost associated with applying to programs varies, depending on the number of programs and specialties applied to by applicants. The AAMC ERAS fee structure can be found on its homepage.

Key Organizations in the ERAS Application and Match Process

There are three primary organizations involved with the ERAS application and Match processes. The organizations with which IMGs must become familiar are:

- Educational Commission for Foreign Medical Graduates (ECFMG)
- Association of American Medical Colleges (AAMC)
- National Resident Matching Program (NRMP)

Each of these organizations is independent of one another and provides primary source information for applicants seeking accurate and up-to-date information about applying and matching to residency training positions. Oftentimes IMGs rely on information provided by friends and colleagues, or they seek guidance through companies soliciting its services to IMGs for additional fees. IMGs should instead go directly to the resource and contact ECFMG, AAMC, or the NRMP as appropriate. An ECFMG representative is available Monday through Friday, 9:00 AM to 5:00 PM Eastern Time, at 215-386-5900; alternatively, IMGs can submit written inquiries by e-mail to eras-support@ecfmg.org. IMGs should visit the Web sites below periodically for up-to-date information:

- www.ecfmg.org/eras
- www.aamc.org/eras
- www.nrmp.com (go to Independent Applicants)
- IMGs may also find it useful to subscribe to the electronic ECFMG ERAS News at (www.ecfmg.org/eras/erasnews.html)

ERAS Support Services at ECFMG

ERAS Support Services provides a number of services to IMGs, including personal in-structional information about the ERAS application process. ERAS Support Services pro-vides IMGs with the following services:

- Client support
- Token issuance
- Document tracking service
- Scanning, uploading, and transmitting of documents to the ERAS PostOffice
- Timeline information
- "Repeat Applicant" services (a service provided to IMGs who participated in the previous ERAS season; see below for details)
- Return of Document Service (RoDS)

Important Note: IMGs already enrolled in U.S. training programs and planning to ap-ply to subspecialty training programs should not request a Token through ECFMG OASIS. All resident physicians in training, IMGs, and U.S. medical graduates must secure a sepa-rate Fellowship Token through the ERAS Fellowships Documents Office (EFDO) at https://www.erasfellowshipdocuments.org/.

ERAS Application and Match Cycle

Table 3-1 lists the schedule of application tasks to be completed during the ERAS Application season. *Dates are subject to change and should be verified directly with the appropriate medical organization/entity.* For complete information, refer to the NRMP Main Match Schedule and the AAMC ERAS Timeline.

ERAS Supporting Documents

The standard document types to be submitted for transmission in support of the ERAS residency application are:

- Original Letters of Recommendation (LORs)
- Original Medical Student Performance Evaluation (formerly referred to as the "Dean's" Letter)
- Medical School Transcripts
- Photograph
- California Application Status Letter (if applying to programs in California)

IMGs are not to submit additional documents for scanning. Oftentimes IMGs will sub-mit their curriculum vitae, ECFMG certificate, passport information, birth certificates, etc. These documents will not be scanned. Should individual programs request additional document types from IMGs, they should make arrangements to forward those documents directly to the requesting programs.

Document Submission Form

An ERAS Document Submission Form must accompany all documents submitted to ERAS Support Services. A new Document Submission Form must be included each time a new document is submitted to ECFMG. Applicants are required to complete the online Document Submission Form located at ECFMG OASIS.

TABLE 3-1

Suggested Schedule for ERAS Application Season

Date	Comments
June	IMGs must update their e-mail and mailing addresses and request ERAS Token using ECFMG's OASIS beginning June 30. Note research programs of interest. IMGs should approach their letter writers now.
June 30	ECFMG begins to generate residency Tokens for IMGs who have made the required payment.
July 1	The AAMC MyERAS Web site opens. Register now.
Mid-July	Once registered at MyERAS, submit supporting documents for scanning to ERAS Support Services at ECFMG in time to arrive on or before August 1.
Mid-August	Registration for the National Resident Matching Program (NRMP), or "the Match", opens on the NRMP Web site. Register now!
First week in September	ERAS PostOffice opens. IMGs can start using the MyERAS site to transmit their Common Application Form (CAF), Profile, and Personal Statement(s) to the ERAS PostOffice. ERAS Support Services at ECFMG starts to transmit supporting documents that have been received and scanned and will continue to scan and transmit documents every business day through May 31. ERAS Support Services will continue to update/transmit ECFMG status reports and USMLE transcripts every business day through the end of May.
Late September	Submit MSPEs in time to arrive at ERAS Support Services at ECFMG on October 1.
October through December	Program directors start their resident selection process and conduct interviews.
November 1	MSPEs are released to programs by the ERAS PostOffice, regardless of when they were originally transmitted to the ERAS PostOffice by ERAS Support Services at ECFMG.
November 30	NRMP Match registration deadline. (Registration after this deadline is available by paying an additional late registration fee to the NRMP.)
Mid-February	NRMP Match late registration deadline. NRMP Match Rank Order List certification deadline.
Mid-March	Applicant matched and unmatched information posted to NRMP Web site. NRMP Post-Match Scramble. Results of Match announced by NRMP.
First week in April	Registration at AAMC MyERAS closes.
May 31	ERAS PostOffice closes, ending current ERAS cycle.
July 1	Residency training begins.

Four-Week Lead Time to Scan and Upload Documents

ERAS Support Services requires a four-week lead time to scan and transmit documents to the ERAS PostOffice due to the large number of IMGs participating in ERAS. IMGs are strongly urged to submit their supporting documents in time to arrive on or before August 1. Because programs currently cannot access MSPEs until November 1, medical schools and IMGs must plan to submit MSPEs in time to arrive by October 1.

Letters of Recommendation (LORs)

LORs are an essential part of the ERAS application and are carefully read by program directors during the resident selection process. An LOR should provide program directors with information on an applicant's clinical abilities, ability to interact with patients and hospital staff, level of professionalism, interpersonal skills, intelligence, level of commitment, and overall qualitative characteristics. LORs act as a forecaster on how successful the student or former graduate will be in the program director's training program. The letter writer should be a faculty member or department head who has evaluated the student or graduate in a clinical setting. IMGs conducting research under the tutelage of a research mentor should remember that the LOR will carry more weight if the research was conducted in the specialty field being pursued in the residency application. Engaging in activities in the specialty of choice, whether it is an elective rotation, observership, or volunteering, is certainly beneficial to an IMG's ERAS application. Program directors also use LORs to discern the commitment level and exposure to the specialty to which applicants are applying.

It is important for IMGs to understand that their ERAS residency application and accompanying LORs are the first presentation made to program directors. In order to make the best possible impression to their applied-to programs, LORs should be up-to-date and meaningful in content. It is reasonable for recent medical school graduates to submit LORs that were secured during the final years of medical school. However, letters dated five to seven years from the date of applying to programs or obtained in the first or second year of medical school may be considered to be outdated and of little value.

Another common phenomenon is the submission of handwritten LORs and/or using the same content for letters from various physicians within the same practice. A program director would rather evaluate two or three meaningful LORs rather than several "form" letters that place little or no value on the IMG's residency application. In all cases, it is important to keep in mind that program directors are interested in receiving information on an applicant's current clinical skill set and qualitative characteristics. Therefore IMGs are urged to submit original LORs that are current, meaningful, and substantive in content.

ECFMG's Original Document Policy

In June 2006 ECFMG implemented an "original document" policy requiring all international medical students and graduates to submit original Letters of Recommendation (LORs) and Medical Student Performance Evaluation (MSPE) in support of their ERAS application. As stated in the policy, the ECFMG specific requirements are:

■ The LOR must be written on official institutional letterhead and manually signed by the letter writer in an ink color other than black.
■ The MSPE must be written on medical school letterhead with the medical school seal affixed, and signed by the designated medical school official.

The policy further states that the ECFMG conducts a "visual inspection" to determine if the document is an original or a copy. ECFMG does not primary-source verify these supporting ERAS documents. If the document is determined to be a copy based on a "visual inspection", ERAS Support Services at ECFMG will stamp the document(s) to read as follows:

■ COPY—Originals Required For This Document Type
■ ERAS Support Services

The policy was implemented to:

■ Establish consistent standards equal to U.S. medical graduates applying to programs via ERAS

- Enhance the quality of documents presented to program directors
- Increase IMG awareness on the importance of these supporting documents and the evaluation process conducted by program directors

While it is an ECFMG requirement for IMGs to submit original LORs, ERAS Support Services at ECFMG will scan the LOR and/or MSPE with the aforementioned annotation placed on the document if the document submitted is determined to be a copy.

Important Note: Programs are not to disqualify any IMG's ERAS application based solely on an annotated LOR or MSPE, nor should the copy stamp infer "irregular behavior" on the part of the IMG.

Waiving Rights to See the LOR

Letter writers supporting an applicant's residency application by writing an LOR may require the applicant's consent not to view the letter, thus allowing the letter writer to be candid and straightforward. Typically, letter writers will reference in the content of such letters that the applicant waived the right to see the letter. Program directors evaluating "waived rights" LORs generally consider the content to be unbiased. The final decision about waiving the right to see the LOR rests with the applicant. Applicants formally file a written consent to waive their rights to see LORs by completing the AAMC's Request for Letter of Recommendation (LOR) Coversheet and submitting it to the letter writer(s). Upon submission to ERAS Support Services for scanning, the letter writer must include the completed LOR Coversheet and with the ECFMG Document Submission Form provided by the IMG. The LOR Coversheet can be downloaded directly from the MyERAS Web site.

Fraudulent Letters of Recommendation

IMGs should be aware that the submission of fraudulent LORs to ECFMG constitutes irregular behavior, as defined by ECFMG. Allegations of irregular behavior are reviewed by the ECFMG Medical Education Credentials Committee, a standing committee of the ECFMG Board of Trustees. If the Committee determines an individual has engaged in irregular behavior, the following actions will take place:

- A permanent annotation will be included in his or her ECFMG Status Reports and Certification Verification Service (CVS) Reports
- Additional information explaining the basis for the finding of irregular behavior and the resulting action will accompany every ECFMG Status Report and CVS Report and may also be provided to legitimately interested entities
- The decision will be reported to the Federation of State Medical Boards Board Action Data Bank, state medical licensing authorities, directors of graduate medical education programs, and to any other organization or individual who, in the judgment of ECFMG, has a legitimate interest in such information.

Furthermore, ECFMG may:

- Bar an individual from exams
- Withhold or revoke a Standard ECFMG Certificate

In recent years a determination of irregular behavior has been made in 12 cases based upon the submission of either altered or wholly fabricated letters of recommendation. In

11 of these cases, the applicant's Standard ECFMG Certificate was revoked and hence these individuals are not eligible to participate in an accredited GME program nor are they eligible to take USMLE Step 3.

The AAMC ERAS Integrity Promotion Education Program (http://www.aamc.org/students/eras/policies/integritypromotioneducation.htm) defines fraudulent activity constituting irregular behavior as:

- Omission of education extension
- Omission of previous residency training
- Submission of fraudulent publication citations
- Submission of fraudulent LORs
- Plagiarism of personal statements

Medical Student Performance Evaluation (MSPE)

The MSPE, formerly referred to as the "Dean's Letter", is a formal evaluation of the student's performance during his/her medical school career. The MSPE is written by an official at the medical school from which the IMG will or has graduated. The MSPE must be written on medical school letterhead with the medical school seal affixed, and signed by the designated medical school official, in accordance with the aforementioned "Original Document Policy". The MSPE should not attempt to predict the IMG's future performance but should provide information about past academic performance. The medical school official is typically the Dean or Principal of the medical school and is the author of the MSPE. IMGs should approach their designated official to acquire the MSPE. The AAMC has published A *Guide to the Preparation of the Medical Student Performance Evaluation* (www.aamc.org/students/eras/resources/downloads/mspeguide.pdf) for medical school use in developing the MSPE.

It is not a mandatory requirement to secure an MSPE in the exact format suggested in the published guideline, because medical school resources dictate what is achievable. However, ERAS Support Services suggests to international medical schools that they include the six sections as outlined in the guideline. Program directors evaluate the MSPE, particularly extracting information about the student's academic performance, class ranking, continuity of the student's educational pathway, and medical student performance relative to his peers. It is suggested that international medical schools should review the MSPE with their students to discuss their documented academic performance.

ERAS Support Services at ECFMG is aware of difficulties encountered by IMGs in securing MSPEs. To that end, the IMG can opt to select "No" on the last page of the Common Application Form (CAF). A placeholder letter will be provided in lieu of the MSPE to instruct program directors to contact the IMG directly if they have any questions or concerns. The IMG's ERAS application will not be considered "incomplete" if the MSPE cannot be provided; however, it is important to note that the MSPE is valued highly and evaluated carefully by program directors.

One of the common mistakes made by IMGs is the assignment of the MSPE as an LOR. The MSPE is not an LOR and should not be assigned as such. All MSPEs must be submitted to ERAS Support Services at ECFMG in time to arrive by October 1, because there is the four-week lead time to scan and upload documents. Currently the MSPE is released to programs on November 1.

Medical School Transcript

The medical school transcript is another standard document. Copies of medical school transcripts are acceptable as long as they are clear copies with a light background. The medical school transcript allows program directors to evaluate the IMG's coursework and grades. If the IMG cannot provide a medical school transcript, the IMG can select "No" on the last page of the Common Application Form (CAF). A placeholder letter in lieu of the medical school transcript will instruct program directors to contact the IMG if they have any questions or concerns.

Photograph

A photograph is another standard requirement used by programs to identify applicants called in for interviews. ERAS Support Services at ECFMG currently implemented a technical enhancement that allows IMGs to upload a digital photograph via OASIS. Technical requirements are specified at the OASIS Web site and at www.ecfmg.org/eras (click on the "Document" section). ERAS Support Services at ECFMG encourages IMGs to utilize this technical feature; otherwise, a physical photograph must be submitted for manual scanning in accordance with the requirements specified on the ECFMG ERAS homepage.

California Application Status Letter

IMGs planning to apply to programs located in the state of California are required to obtain an Application Status Letter issued by the Medical Board of California, a process that will take several months. This letter verifies that the IMG's medical education has been reviewed and approved as meeting California's licensing requirements. When the IMG lists the names of letter writers in the MyERAS Documents section, IMGs must include as one of their LORs the "California Letter", instead of a letter writer's name. In this case, IMGs can assign up to three LORs and the "California Letter" to any program in California.

USMLE Transcript

The USMLE transcript contains the examinee's entire USMLE history on Step 1, Step 2 CK, Step 2 CS and, if taken, Step 3. It includes all attempts: passed, failed, incomplete, etc. The USMLE transcript will also list any annotations regarding test accommodations, if provided; annotations of information documenting classification of any scores as undefined; any annotations of irregular behavior; and notations of any actions taken against an examinee by medical licensing authorities or other credentialing agencies reported to the Federation of State Medical Boards (FSMB).

The USMLE transcript is not transmitted automatically. IMGs may request its transmission, and are highly encouraged to do so, to their applied-to programs and pay a one-time fee. IMGs can request a USMLE transcript from the Documents tab of MyERAS.

ECFMG Status Report

ERAS Support Services at ECFMG automatically transmits the IMG's ECFMG Status Report to all applied-to programs without any additional costs. The ECFMG Status Report is a document issued by ECFMG verifying the IMG's ECFMG certification status. The ECFMG Status Report does not contain scores and does not indicate the number of attempts made to take the examination. For any IMG who received an FSMB Board

Action Report, the Board Action Report will be attached directly onto the IMG's ECFMG Status Report and made viewable to program directors.

Repeat Applicants and Automatic Uploading of Documents

"Repeat ERAS Applicants" are defined as IMGs who participated in the previous ERAS application season and will participate in the upcoming ERAS application season. "Repeat ERAS Applicants" will be identified at the time they make an ERAS Token request via ECFMG OASIS. ERAS Support Services will retrieve their stored MSPEs, medical school transcripts, and photographs and upload them to the ERAS PostOffice, if submitted in the previous year, within three to five business days from the time the IMG uses the Token to register at MyERAS.

Any IMG identified as a "Repeat ERAS Applicant" is not required to resubmit the MSPE, medical school transcript, or photograph unless any one of these document types has been updated. Retrieval of stored documents is only available to IMGs who applied the immediately previous year, not in earlier years.

"Repeat ERAS Applicants" are required to submit their LORs. It is highly discouraged to re-use these documents year after year. Program directors are only interested in the IMG's current clinical activities.

OASIS Online Document Tracking System

ERAS Support Services provides IMGs with receipt confirmation of all document types submitted for scanning by posting the receipt date and document type to their ECFMG OASIS account. ERAS Support Services at ECFMG also publishes the date documents are scanned for transmission to the ERAS PostOffice. The "scan date" is published on the ERAS homepage.

Return of Document Service (RODS)

For IMGs who want to have their ERAS supporting documents returned to them, ERAS Support Services provides a Return of Document Service (RODS). This service allows IMGs to request the return of ERAS eligible documents, via ECFMG OASIS. Letters of recommendation for which the right to see has been waived cannot be returned. Use of RODS requires a nominal payment of the posted fee plus the cost for courier service.

AAMC MyERAS On-line Application Process

THE COMMON APPLICATION FORM (CAF)

The on-line Common Application Form (CAF), which all applicants applying to programs must complete and submit, can be accessed at the MyERAS Web site. The CAF essentially serves as the applicant's curriculum vitae, and applicants cannot apply to programs until it is certified and submitted.

Some tips for completing the CAF:

- Use the worksheet provided by the AAMC.
- Make sure all information is accurate, honest, and consistent with other documented entries.
- Leave any field blank if the question is not applicable.

Once the CAF is completed, carefully review all information for accuracy. *Once the CAF is certified, it cannot be changed or updated.*

PERSONAL STATEMENTS

Applicants applying to residency training programs have the ability to create one or more on-line personal statements at the MyERAS Web site. Applicants may craft personal statements to be assigned and sent to individual programs.

■ A personal statement is also particularly helpful in conveying to programs any specific visa or U.S. pending permanent resident status information. For example, IMGs requiring visas should clarify their current immigration status and the expected visa type(s) they hope to secure through the prospective training program. However, it is important for IMGs who may need a visa to research those institutions that assist and are familiar with the visa processes.

■ If a program requires information that is not included in your transcript or CAF, students and graduates may create a personal statement including these details and assign it to that specific program.

■ Create a personal statement(s) using a word processor to perform a spell check. A well-written, error-free personal statement is necessary if an IMG is serious about making a good impression on program directors.

■ There are a number of Web sites that contain examples of personal statements. Do not cut and paste any information found at these sites into your statement. This action is deemed as plagiarism. For more information, go to www.aamc.org/students/eras/policies/integrityeducation.htm.

NRMP MATCH

Purpose of the Match

The National Resident Matching Program (NRMP) is a private, not-for-profit corporation that provides a uniform date of appointment to positions in graduate medical education (GME). The NRMP is not an application processing service; rather, it provides an impartial venue for matching applicants' and programs' preferences for each other consistently.

The purpose of the Match is to assist applicants in obtaining GME positions in the program of their highest preference while helping programs recruit applicants whom they have deemed most desirable. As such, the goal is to optimize the match of applicant and program. The Match cannot ensure that an applicant receives a position in his or her first-choice program but will match the applicant with the program that has expressed a desire to recruit that applicant as close to their first choice as possible.

In contrast to the processes before the establishment of the Match, the uniform appointment date now precludes frustrating rounds of negotiations in which applicants may be offered multiple positions but in a sequence and time frame that might force premature commitment and subsequent regret on the part of both the applicant and the program.

Although virtually all programs that participate in the Match also participate in ERAS, these are two distinct programs. Applicants must apply to both in order to participate in both.

Participation

Students or graduates of international medical schools listed in IMED are eligible to participate in the Match. The process begins by registering with the NRMP. This can be done online at www.nrmp.org, but before registering it is important that applicants carefully read the Match Participation Agreement on the site to be clear with respect to their obligations and restrictions as participants as well as those of the participating programs.

The NRMP R3 (Registration, Ranking, Results) system requires an AAMC ID number, which will be issued in the process of registration. Applicants will be asked to create a personal password and to select which of the Independent Applicant Types describes their medical training. For IMGs, that will be either U.S. citizen or non-U.S. citizen graduate/student of an international medical school. In addition, IMGs must submit their USMLE/ECFMG identification number.

Note that to participate in the Match, IMGs need not be medical school graduates nor must they have achieved ECFMG certification. However, they must have passed all required examinations for ECFMG certification (USMLE Step 1, Step 2 CK and Step 2 CS), and results must be available by the Rank Order List (ROL) deadline (see below). There are some older examinations that may satisfy requirements. Information about the NRMP examination requirements to participate in the Match can be found at www.nrmp.org. Registration may be initiated before the examination results are available, but if they are not available by the ROL deadline, the registrant will be automatically withdrawn from the Match.

It is critical for applicants to enter their names accurately and be certain their entry is identical to the name as entered in the ERAS application. They will also be asked to select the name of their medical school from a drop-down list and enter the month and year of their actual or expected graduation date.

The registration fee must be paid electronically at the time of registration. Note that late registration (after November 30) requires an additional fee. The registration fee allows the applicant to rank as many as 20 programs on their primary rank order list. Applicants may also submit supplemental rank order list(s) only if they have ranked advanced (PGY-2) positions on their primary rank order lists and wish, in addition, to secure a first-year (PGY-1) position. Again, listing up to 20 programs on the supplemental rank order list is covered by the basic registration fee. Additional programs can be added to either the primary or supplemental rank order lists at an additional cost per program. Note that all fees are subject to change; the NRMP Web site should be consulted for current fees.

Creating the Rank Order List

NRMP provides a downloadable worksheet on its site that applicants are encouraged to complete before entering ranks into the R3 System. Applicants should enter the exact name of the Sponsoring Institution and the Program/Description as well as the Type of Program and the program's NRMP Program Code. Then rank order numbers can be assigned and/or modified prior to entry.

In addition to being sure that the program is of the right specialty and at an institution acceptable to the applicant, it is important to be sure that the program is of the correct type for the applicant. There are four types of programs that may participate in the Match, although only three are available to IMGs.

Categorical programs begin in the PGY-1 year, whereas *advanced programs* begin in the PGY-2 year after a year of prerequisite training. Residents accepted into these programs can expect to advance through the full program without need for reapplication each year, assuming satisfactory progress. Both types of programs provide the training required for board certification in medical specialties.

In contrast, *preliminary programs* are PGY-1 year programs of only one year's duration and include Preliminary Medicine programs, Preliminary Surgery programs, and Transitional programs. While the first two primarily serve to provide prerequisite training for advanced programs, Transitional programs do not as clearly qualify participants for entry into Advanced programs, and IMGs on J-1 or H-1B visas may have difficulty continuing their training after the Transitional year. For that reason, they should think carefully before ranking such programs unless they have viable options to continue training beyond that year. Also, these programs by themselves will not qualify participants to sit for medical specialty board examinations.

Whenever a list is submitted it must be certified by the applicant for use in the actual Match. At any time prior to the RoL deadline, previously submitted lists may be altered or substituted, but each time the final version must be certified by the applicant.

Note the following from the NRMP Web site: "Applicants should list programs in their actual order of preference, beginning with rank #1 for the most preferred program. Their choices should not be influenced by speculation about whether a particular program will rank them high, low, or not at all. The position of a program on an applicant's rank order list will not affect the applicant's position on a program's rank order list. Applicants must not rank any programs they are unwilling to attend."

Factors driving applicant ranking of programs certainly include choice of specialty, training institution, and location, but it is also necessary to consider how competitive each program is and to be realistic about the strength of the applicant's application. Certainly experience and impressions gained during an interview should weigh heavily, although implications about the program's intention to rank the applicants should not be overweighted and may in fact be in conflict with NRMP's policy on persuasion (see below). NRMP has tracked the length of the RoLs of both applicants and programs over the past several years and found a positive correlation (i.e., applicants who match tend to have ranked more programs than those who do not match). Other than cost beyond the first 20 programs ranked, there is no disadvantage to including more programs on a rank order list, but there is one strong caveat: *Applicants should never list a program that they are not willing to enter, because under the terms of the Match they are legally bound to any program with which they match.*

Applicants may begin registration in mid-August but must complete registration before the end of November to avoid the late registration fee. Final rank order lists can be entered beginning in mid-January but must be submitted and certified by the last Wednesday in February. The actual calendar dates for each annual cycle are posted on the NRMP Web site.

How the Match Works

Concurrent with Match applicants creating and submitting their rank order list of preferred programs, programs are also submitting a rank order list of preferred applicants. Programs rank applicants based on complete review of their ERAS materials as well as their impressions at the time of interview. Just as applicants should never rank programs that they would never want to join, programs never rank applicants that they do not want. Generally speaking, programs will rarely if ever rank applicants who have not been interviewed.

The NRMP Match Participation Agreement, which all applicants must agree to, is very clear on communications between applicants and programs prior to the Match. The following sections address this topic.

Restrictions on Persuasion

One of the purposes of the Matching Program is to allow both applicants and programs to make selection decisions on a uniform schedule and without undue or unwarranted pressure. Both applicants and programs may express a high degree of interest in each other and try to encourage future ranking decisions in their favor but must not solicit statements implying a commitment. Although applicants and programs may volunteer how they plan to rank each other, "it is a breach of this Agreement to request such information. In addition, only the final preferences of programs and applicants, as expressed on their final certified rank order lists, will determine the offering of positions and the placement of applicants through the Matching Program. It is a breach of this Agreement for a participant in the Matching Program to make any verbal or written contract for appointment to a concurrent year residency position prior to the Matching Program."

It is quite acceptable and probably good practice for applicants to notify their most preferred programs that they intend to rank them highly, and many programs will often similarly notify their most desirable applicants. However, these communications must never cross the line into actual or implied commitments.

The Match uses a complex algorithm to sort through tens of thousands of rank order lists to find the optimal match of applicant and program. An excellent illustration of how the algorithm works can be found on the NRMP Web site. A hypothetical set of applicants and programs is followed step-by-step, with comments on which applicants are using the Match most effectively and appropriately. It is highly worthwhile reviewing this algorithm as well as the many other pages and frequently asked questions (FAQs) on the site. Because the Match may well determine an IMG's entire medical career, it would be prudent to be well versed in its operations and get any questions answered before committing to participation.

On Monday of Match Week, all participating applicants can go to the NRMP Web site and learn whether they have matched or not. At this point applicants who successfully matched will not yet know to which program they have matched but only that they have a position. Applicants who have submitted supplemental rank order lists will also be advised of their status with respect to both their primary and supplemental lists. Some applicants may learn that they have matched on one or the other of their lists but not both, in which case they are considered to be partially matched.

The Scramble

The following day, a list of the location and number of positions available in unfilled programs, the Dynamic List of Unfilled Programs, is posted (and updated hourly). Now unmatched and partially matched applicants may participate in "The Scramble". This refers to the process whereby these applicants may apply directly to unfilled programs in an attempt to secure positions. Match participants who have also been registered participants in ERAS may use ERAS to forward application materials to as many as 30 additional programs that have unfilled positions and up to 15 previously applied-to programs if listed as an unfilled position. See the page entitled "Preparing for the Scramble" on the ERAS section of the AAMC Web site and the ERAS section above. Prior to requesting that materials be sent to the program, applicants should communicate directly by telephone or e-mail to the program indicating their interest in seeking a position through the Scramble. At that point a program may express interest in reviewing the application or may indicate that submission of materials would be pointless, in which case the program should not be pursued. Programs have expressed great annoyance at receiving large numbers of pro forma faxes and e-mail from scrambling applicants. Although time is certainly of the essence, it is still important to convey a personal interest in each program and present as positively as possible.

Thursday of Match Week is Match Day, when results for all matched applicants are posted on the NRMP Web site, including identifying exactly to which program the applicant has matched. The following day, programs send two copies of letters of appointment to their matched applicants. The applicant should sign one copy and return it to the program as soon as possible in order to certify his or her match to the position.

The San Francisco Match

A number of highly competitive specialties, including ophthalmology and plastic surgery, with limited numbers of training positions, participate in a separate match, the San Francisco Match. This match also serves a number of similar fellowships. Information on the current status of the San Francisco Match can be found at www.sfmatch.org.

Positions Outside the Match

Although the vast majority of residency positions are offered through the NRMP Match, some programs choose to offer some or all of their positions to applicants outside of the Match. These offers are usually made after the applicant has interviewed with the program and the program is favorably enough impressed that they want to ensure the applicant will enter their program. These offers can be made to applicants who are currently registered in the Match. However, if such an offer is accepted the applicant must immediately withdraw from the Match.

Deciding whether to accept such an offer can be very difficult and stressful, and there are several issues that must be carefully considered. Although acceptance ensures the applicant a position, it may not be in a preferred program. Accepting such an offer and signing a contract legally binds the applicant to stay with that position, and he or she may not subsequently accept another position offer even if it clearly seems more desirable. Program directors who make offers outside the Match often place short time constraints on the applicant's decision. In addition, until there is a signed contract, the offer and its acceptance continue to be tentative and could be withdrawn. So it was in large part to eliminate the stress and uncertainty of dealing with such offers and to "level the playing field" that the NRMP Match was established. When initially contacting programs and trying to obtain interviews, it is quite reasonable for applicants to inquire as to the program's policy with respect to the Match. It is more difficult to ascertain the significance of a program's offering positions outside the Match because there may be many reasons why they may choose to do so. Again, this is a legitimate question to be raised during an interview.

Before signing contracts outside the Match:

- Make sure the program is one in which you really want to get your training.
- Be sure to distinguish between a letter of agreement and a contract. A letter of agreement is not legally binding, so insist on a formal contract as soon as possible. Do not decline any other options until a contract is signed.

■ You must not sign multiple contracts or even letters of agreement. Program directors who identify applicants making multiple simultaneous commitments may withdraw their offers.

■ You must withdraw from the Match as soon as possible once you sign a contract or accept a letter of agreement.

References

■ **American Academy of Family Physicians.** "Tips on Letters of Reference." Strolling Through the Match. Available at www.aafp.org/online/en/home/publications/otherpubs/strolling/prep/lettersreference.html. Accessed 19 December 2007.

■ **Hart R.** Effective Networking for Professional Success: Making the Most of Your Personal Contacts (Better Management Skills Series). New York: Stirling Books; 1996.

■ **Wright SM, Zeigelstein RC.** Writing more-informative letters of reference. J Gen Intern Med. 2004;19:588–93.

4 Transitioning to the United States

Eleanor M. Fitzpatrick, MA, and Tracy Wallowicz

Visa Issues   58

Visitor Visas   58

- Initial Visa Application Process   59
- Visa Options for GME Training   60

J-1 Visa Sponsorship for GME Training   60

H-1B Visa for GME Training   62

- Implications of Personal and Professional Difficulties During GME Training   64
- Maintaining Visa Status   64

Other Logistical Issues Relating to Travel   65

Initial Entry into the United States   65

Summary   65

Visa Issues

Understanding and complying with immigration guidelines is critical for foreign national physicians interested in pursuing GME training in the United States. U.S. immigration law is governed by specific federal regulations defined in the Immigration and Nationality Act (INA). The entry and monitoring of foreign nationals in the United States is coordinated through strict inter-agency coordination among various branches of the Department of Homeland Security (DHS) and the Department of State (DoS) (Table 4-1).

TABLE 4-1

Roles of Department of State (DoS) & Department of Homeland Security (DHS) in Visa Oversight

Bureaus within Department of Homeland Security (DHS) Responsible for Immigration Policies, Procedures, and Enforcement	Bureaus within Department of State (DoS) Responsible for Management of Visa Processes
■ U.S. Customs and Border Protection (CBP): security of America's borders	■ Bureau of Educational and Cultural Affairs: oversight of all Exchange Visitor Programs
■ U.S. Immigration and Custom Enforcement (ICE): investigations, detention, removal, intelligence, SEVIS	■ Bureau of Consular Affairs: U.S. consulate review of visa eligibility
■ U.S. Citizenship and Immigration Services (CIS): adjudications previously performed by INS	

In reviewing visa issues as they relate to foreign national physicians, it is important to be familiar with the terms *visa* and *visa status*.

A *visa* is a permit issued by an official at a U.S. consulate or embassy abroad that is stamped on or affixed to the passport. The visa represents the approval to seek entry to the United States for a specific purpose and related immigration classification (e.g., B-1/B-2 Visitor, J-1 exchange visitor physician, H-1B temporary specialty worker).

Visa status reflects the specific legal classification in which the foreign national is formally admitted into the United States. It also denotes the duration of approved stay. Visa status is confirmed by a Customs and Border Patrol (CBP) officer at the port-of-entry for an initial entry or by the regional service center officer of U.S. Citizenship and Immigration Services (USCIS) for those who seek a change of status after arrival. All foreign nationals must abide by the terms and dates of the visa status noted on the I-94 card, Arrival/Departure Record or Notice of Action.

VISITOR VISAS

For many foreign national physicians, their initial introduction to the U.S. immigration system occurs when they apply for a visa to come to the United States to take the USMLE Step 2 Clinical Skills (CS) examination, to interview with GME programs, and/or to participate in clinical observerships. Most foreign national physicians who enter the United States for these purposes do so on visitors' visas (B-1 for "business" or B-2 for "tourism"). However, citizens from some designated countries may be admitted to the U.S for up to 90 days without a visa under a special visa waiver program (see http://travel.state.gov/visa/temp/without/without_1990.html). In all cases, physicians who enter the country as temporary visitors must be prepared to document the purpose of travel, the proposed length of stay, and a clear intent to return to the home country or country of last legal permanent residence.

When preparing to visit the United States, physicians must compile all official documentation related to their planned activities. Such documents must include, but may not be limited to, the items listed in Box 4-1.

☑ **BOX 4-1   Documentation for Planned Trip to the United States**

- Step 2 CS and/or Step 3 registration and confirmation
- Confirmation letters for interviews
- Certification of current school enrollment and/or employment in one's home country
- Any other medical credentials
- A return airline ticket
- Financial records
- Confirmation letter for physician or medical student for preapproved participation in clinical observerships or clerkships at U.S. academic medical centers

---

Initial Visa Application Process

As a general rule, all nonimmigrant visa applicants are required to appear for a personal interview at a U.S. embassy or consulate presumably in one's home country. Scheduling the initial visa interview and then waiting for the security clearance can take months. Therefore, preparation and planning is essential. Foreign national physicians or medical students are advised to contact the consulate well in advance for information on scheduling times and specific application requirements (Box 4-2).

☑ **BOX 4-2   Initial Visa Application Process Requirements**

- Form DS-156, "Application for Nonimmigrant Visa"
- Form DS-157, "Supplemental Application for Nonimmigrant Visa"
- Biometric finger printing
- Fees
- Name checks
- Security clearances

Web sites for U.S. embassies and consulates can be found on the DoS homepage at http://usembassy.state.gov. Timelines for visa appointments and general processing information can be found at http://travel.state.gov/visa/temp/wait/tempvisitors_wait.php.

A B-1 or B-2 visitor visa restricts a foreign national to participation in non-paid activities and is limited to a maximum stay of six months, based on the discretion of the reviewing customs officer. Upon arrival to the United States, a port-of-entry official reviews the individual's proposed plan, financial information, etc. and determines an appropriate end date of authorized stay. The date is marked on the individual's I-94 card (Arrival/Departure Record). Foreign national physicians and medical students must be extremely careful not to violate the terms of their visa status or overstay the dates of authorized stay as marked on the I-94 card. There are serious penalties for visa violations and overstays which can negatively impact one's future immigration options.

Visa Options for GME Training

Foreign national physicians who secure contracts for U.S. GME positions must obtain an appropriate visa prior to beginning the training program. There are various temporary, non-immigrant visa options available for GME training. The most common include the J-1 "Exchange Visitor" physician category and the H-1 B "Temporary Worker in a Specialty Occupation".

Foreign national physicians may also qualify to train as medical residents/fellows with a valid employment authorization document (EAD). The USCIS grants this work authorization in conjunction with a variety of immigrant and non-immigrant petitions (e.g., F-1 Student on Optional Practical Training (OPT), J-2, dependent of a J-1 principle, family of a U.S. citizen or legal permanent resident, refugee or asylee status). In exceptional cases, foreign national physicians may also qualify for O-1 visas that are reserved for "Individuals of Extraordinary Ability". The O-1 visa requires superior credentials and documented international renown and, therefore, is rarely used for GME training purposes.

Teaching hospitals, like all U.S. employers, are responsible for complying with federal guidelines associated with the hiring of non-U.S. citizens. Immigration and employment laws mandate that teaching hospitals pay certain filing fees and assume administrative oversight of foreign national physicians participating in their GME programs. It is not uncommon for hospitals to limit the types of visas (e.g., only J-1 or only H-1B) they will accept for trainees enrolling in their programs. Foreign national physicians are advised to inquire about the immigration options offered by the programs they are considering prior to filing initial residency applications. It is important to clearly understand specific regulatory requirements, restrictions, costs, timelines, and institutional policies that apply to the various visa/immigration options.

J-1 VISA SPONSORSHIP FOR GME TRAINING

Historically, the J-1 has been the most common visa classification used for foreign national physicians in GME training. The J-1 is a temporary nonimmigrant visa reserved for participants in the Exchange Visitor Program. As a public diplomacy initiative of the DoS, the Exchange Visitor Program was established to enhance international exchange and mutual understanding between the people of the United States and other nations. In keeping with the Program's goals for international education, J-1 physicians are required to return home for at least two years following their training before being eligible for certain U.S. visas. Exceptions can be made in the case of waivers (see below).

The DoS designated the ECFMG as the sole visa sponsor for all J-1 physicians who participate in clinical training programs. ECFMG administers its sponsorship program in accordance with the provisions of the DoS and federal regulations. ECFMG is responsible for ensuring that J-1 physicians and teaching institutions meet the federal requirements for participation. ECFMG does not sponsor physicians for other U.S. visa types.

Foreign national physicians who seek J-1 sponsorship to enter graduate medical education (GME) programs must fulfill a number of general requirements as detailed in the application materials published by ECFMG. See Box 4-3 for the minimum J-1 requirements a physician applicant must have.

The current requirements for ECFMG certification ensure that J-1 physicians have "adequate prior education and training to participate satisfactorily in the program for which they are coming to the United States" and have "competency in oral and written English." The current ECFMG Certification requirements (see Chapter 2) include the primary

---

✓ BOX 4-3 **Minimum J-1 Visa Requirements**

■ Adequate prior education/training and English competency
■ ECFMG certification
■ Statement of Need from the Ministry of Health
■ Contract for a GME position

---

source verification of the final medical diploma and transcript by ECFMG with the medical school and passing scores on the USMLE Step 1, Step 2 CK, and Step 2 CS.

J-1 physician applicants must also provide ECFMG with a Statement of Need from the central office of the Ministry of Health of the country of most recent legal permanent residence. The Statement of Need, which follows specific regulatory language, documents the home government's support for the specific training that the J-1 physician will pursue and confirms the physician's intent to return to home to practice medicine upon completion of training in the United States. The Statement of Need is consistent with the compulsory obligation of the two-year home residence requirement for all J-1 physicians, and their J-2 dependents. The home residence requirement requires that J-1 physicians and accompanying J-2 dependents reside in the home country for an aggregate of at least two years before being eligible for certain changes or adjustment in visa status in the United States. Various legal options have evolved to allow J-1 physicians to waive the return home obligation, the most common being employment in a U.S. medically underserved area (MUA) or Health Professions Shortage Area (HPSA).

J-1 sponsorship for GME training is dependent on a contract or official letter of offer for a GME position. Each J-1 physician applicant must secure the training contract prior to applying to ECFMG for visa sponsorship. ECFMG is authorized to sponsor physicians for training in base residencies and subspecialty fellowships that are accredited by the Accreditation Council for Graduate Medical Education (ACGME) as well as for some advanced non-standard fellowships. J-1 sponsorship is generally issued in increments of one year in conjunction with the GME academic year of July 1 through June 30 and so must be renewed annually.

Once a physician has been approved for J-1 sponsorship, ECFMG creates an electronic record for the physician in the Student Exchange Visitor Information System (SEVIS) and issues Forms DS-2019, "Certificate of Eligibility for Exchange Visitor (J-1) Status". Through an interagency partnership between DoS and DHS, SEVIS tracks and monitors the activities of all J-1 visa holders. A foreign national physician with an active SEVIS record and an original Form DS-2019 may apply for J-1 visa and/or visa status from agencies of the U.S. Government.

J-1 physicians may request ECFMG sponsorship for dependent spouses and minor children. The J-2 spouse may seek employment authorization through USCIS to work in any position for which they are qualified, including GME training. The duration of stay for the J-2 is limited to the approved timeline for the J-1 principal and cannot be extended independent of the primary visa holder.

J-1 physicians are responsible to comply with all U.S. laws and regulations pertaining to foreign nationals. Various regulations govern the scope, pathway, and duration of the activities pursued by a J-1 physician. The scope of training and employment authorization derived from J-1 visa sponsorship is specific to the training proposal approved by ECFMG. J-1 physicians are specifically prohibited from employment outside of their GME program. This prohibition includes moonlighting (i.e., paid clinical work beyond the core requirements of the GME program whether in the institution sponsoring GME or elsewhere) (see Chapter 7).

J-1 physicians must pursue a predefined, progressive educational pathway. ECFMG sponsors J-1 physicians for medical specialty training at the base residency level through subspecialty training in advanced fellowships. J-1 physicians are permitted to change specialty once within the first two years of sponsorship. A request to change medical specialty requires reestablishing eligibility for sponsorship, including confirmation that the proposed training can be completed within the maximum duration of participation. J-1 physicians are eligible for a maximum of 7 years of training, provided that they are progressing in an approved GME program. The duration of sponsorship is directly linked to the standard board certification requirements as established by the member boards of the American Board of Medical Specialties (ABMS) and/or the ACGME-accredited length of the program. J-1 sponsorship can be extended briefly to remain in the United States for an ABMS-member board certification exam.

To ensure strict regulatory compliance, the J-1 visa sponsorship process requires close coordination between the teaching institution, the physician applicant and ECFMG. Each academic institution designates a Training Program Liaison (TPL) to serve as the official representative to communicate with ECFMG regarding all J-1 matters. TPLs can be the source of a great deal of assistance and information, and J-1 physicians should establish good working relationships with their TPL at each program in which they enroll throughout the duration of their ECFMG-sponsored training.

H-1B Visa for GME Training

The H-1B visa is reserved for temporary workers in specialty occupations who hold professional degrees. Today, the H-1B is offered by many institutions for GME training. In addition to a medical degree and a valid ECFMG certificate, foreign national physicians who are interested in applying for H-1B visas must pass USMLE Step 3 and qualify for the appropriate medical license in the state where the training will take place. Competency in English is also required for the H-1B. Passing USMLE Step 2 CS satisfies the language requirements as the clinical skills exam includes an assessment of spoken English.

The H-1B work/training authorization is employer-specific and requires visa sponsorship directly through the teaching hospital. To sponsor a qualified foreign national physician for a GME position on an H-1B visa, the teaching hospital must file petitions with both the USCIS and the Department of Labor (DoL). The petitions require detailed information about the position being offered including program, location, wage rate and contract dates as well as evidence of the credentials of the individual applicant. Additionally, the sponsoring hospital must confirm that the foreign national will be paid the appropriate salary for the position. As the prospective employer, the teaching hospital must incur certain filing fees associated with the H-1B petitions and must also agree to cover the return home transportation costs, in the unlikely event that the physician be dismissed from the training program before the official end day.

The maximum duration of continuous training/employment in H-1B status is 6 years in most cases. Petitions are approved based on the length of the training contract, not to exceed three years at one time. An approved H-1B petition cannot be transferred for use at another institution, program, or position. The H-1B physician may seek to change positions or transfer to a different hospital/employer; however, a new petition may be required. Mandatory reporting and periodic updates on H-1B physicians is required.

An H-1B physician may have dependent spouse and children accompany them to the U.S. in H-4 status. There is no independent work authorization granted to H-4 dependents; however, participation in educational studies is permitted. The duration of legal stay for the H-4 dependent is directly tied to the timeline of the H-1B principal.

Unlike the J-1, the H-1B visa does not impose a mandatory home residency requirement or a service obligation. Therefore, foreign national physicians who train on H-1B visas may be eligible, in some cases, to pursue direct steps toward permanent resident status (Tables 4-2 and 4-3).

TABLE 4-2

J-1 and H-1B Visas for GME Training

	J-1 Visa	H-1B Visa
Regulatory oversight	Departments of State & Homeland Security, ECFMG	Departments of Labor & Homeland Security
Exams	USMLE Steps 1, 2CK, 2CS	USMLE Steps 1, 2CK, 2CS, 3
Time limit	7 years maximum	6 years maximum
Funding	Multiple sources acceptable	U.S. employer salary only
Home country requirements	Strong ties to home country, 2-year home rule	None
Employment for spouse?	Yes; J-2 can apply for work authorization	No; no work permit for H-4

TABLE 4-3

Documentation Typically Required When Applying for J-1 or H-1B Visa

J-1 Visa	H-1B Visa
■ Form DS-2019, Certificate of Eligibility, signed in blue ink by the Regional Advisor at ECFMG, with a future expiration/end date	■ Original Form I-797, Notice of Action issued by U.S. Citizenship and Immigration Services. showing approval of an H-1B petition, with a future expiration/end date
■ Form DS-158, Contact Information and Work History for Nonimmigrant Visa Applicant	■ Copy of H-1B petition filed by employer on physician's behalf (in some cases only a copy of the Form I-129 petition and Labor Condition Application may be sufficient; check with consulate)
■ Form DS-156, Application for Nonimmigrant Visa, with photos	■ Form DS-156, Application for Nonimmigrant Visa, with photos
■ Form DS-157, Supplemental Nonimmigrant Visa Application (generally required of all male applicants between the ages of 16 and 45)	■ Form DS-157, Supplemental Nonimmigrant Visa Application (generally required of all male applicants between the ages of 16 and 45)
■ Valid passport	■ Valid passport
■ Application and reciprocity fees (check with consulate for fee amounts and how they must be paid)	■ Application and reciprocity fees (check with consulate for fee amounts and how they must be paid)
■ SEVIS fee, if applying for a J-1 visa to begin a new program	—
■ Documents that demonstrate nonimmigrant intent (i.e., proof of intent to return home)	—

Implications of Personal and Professional Difficulties During GME Training

In general, foreign national physicians enrolled in GME training face similar personal and professional challenges as their U.S. citizen counterparts. Health, family, and marital issues, as well as personnel or academic difficulties, can result in an interruption or even termination of a resident's contract. In addition to the emotional, professional, and financial concerns tied to such challenges, foreign national physicians whose visa status is based on enrollment in medical residencies must be keenly aware of the immigration implications of diverting from pre-approved activities and timelines. U.S. immigration regulations and labor laws are not entirely consistent. Therefore, careful review of the nuances of each status is required. Foreign national physicians must be careful to maintain continuous training and immigration records.

Requests for leaves of absence, changes to part-time status, resignations from training, and so on must be pre-approved by the visa sponsor (ECFMG for J-1s, teaching hospitals for H-1Bs, O-1s, etc.). No change should be made without first verifying permissibility of altering the approved educational plan and then clarifying the necessary steps to return to GME training in the future, should that be the physician's intent. Official termination from a GME position may require prompt departure from the United States. In such cases, physicians should contact the visa sponsor for instructions and may also want to consult with an immigration attorney.

A request to transfer institutions for any reason while under active contract requires a formal release from the current program. Eligibility to accept a second offer and apply for a transfer is contingent upon release from the original program. For immigration purposes, it is essential to coordinate a seamless transfer to avoid any gap in training dates. When considering fellowship training or practice options, including J-1 waiver positions. (For in-depth discussion of J-1 visa waivers, see R. Aronson, "Immigration Overview for International Medical Graduates," *State Medical Licensure Requirements and Statistics*. AMA: Chicago; 2004:97-8.) Foreign national physicians are warned against making multiple commitments. Misrepresenting one's intentions or inaccurately reporting one's immigration status or eligibility could be considered a legal or ethical violation and cause long-term negative consequences for physicians.

Maintaining Visa Status

In addition to meeting the academic standards required to progress through GME, foreign national physicians must maintain valid visa status in order to continue to train at

---

☑ **BOX 4-4   Maintaining Visa Status**

- Active participation in approved training program: specific site, salary, dates, etc.
  - J-1 physicians must maintain full-time status in the program
  - Unauthorized employment is considered a violation of status (including moonlighting)
- Possession of required documents/records confirming visa status:
  - For J-1: DS-2019; for H-1B: I-797 with valid dates
  - I-94 record with "Duration of Status" (D/S) or future end-date
  - Valid passport
- Compliance with all reporting requirements
  - Reporting U.S. residential address to U.S. Government (Form AR-11) within 10 days of any move
  - Notification to appropriate offices (i.e., ECFMG, TPL, GME program director, U.S. Government) of proposed changes in location or course of training, leaves of absences, terminations, extensions, etc.
  - Complying with any special registration requirement as instructed by a U.S. government official at port-of-entry, etc.
- Strict adherence to all applicable U.S. laws and regulations

U.S. teaching hospitals. Maintaining status requires, but is not limited to, the items listed in Box 4-4.

Other Logistical Issues Relating to Travel

Foreign national physicians are not required to travel outside the United States every year in order to apply for a new visa. The visa stamp in the passport serves as a permit for a foreign national to enter the United States. The visa stamp can expire after the individual arrives, and the foreign national may legally remain in the United States provided she or he complies with the terms, obligations and dates of the "visa status" as noted above (e.g., J-1, H-1B). However, it is important to note that a foreign national who departs the United States is required to have a valid visa stamp in the passport to be eligible to return. Visas are only issued at U.S. consulates/embassies abroad.

Since a new visa is needed for re-entry, it is not advisable for foreign national physicians with expired visas and/or those who changed visa status within the United States to travel internationally during the training year. Current U.S. visa application processes can involve long waits for consular appointments and security clearances. At present, there is no expedited processing available for background checks. Therefore, it is very hard to guarantee timely return to the training program.

Foreign national physicians who must travel outside the United States are advised to review the dates and purpose of their travel with the GME program director(s) and administrative staff prior to finalizing their plans. A discussion about potential delays and contract provisions for making up lost time, for example, should take place before departure. Physicians should also contact the specific the U.S. embassy or consulate where they intend to apply for the visa to inquire about application procedures, documentation, requirements, and timeframes. It is critical for foreign national physicians (and dependents) to be aware of the documents that will be required for re-entry to the United States. Additional information on travel is available on the ECFMG Web site at http://www.ecfmg.org/evsp/travel.html.

INITIAL ENTRY INTO THE UNITED STATES

Foreign nationals initially entering the US on J-1 visas may enter the country up to 30 days before the start of their contract. However, those on H-1B visas may not enter the country until 10 days before their contract start date.

Summary

Immigration is one of many variables to consider when selecting a U.S. GME program. Foreign national physicians are encouraged to research their visa options very carefully. Institutional policies, procedures, budgets, and deadlines vary widely among teaching hospitals and even among programs within the same institution. Ultimately, the foreign national physician enrolled in U.S. GME training must understand, respect, and comply thoroughly with all U.S. immigration laws and institutional guidelines.

References

- ECFMG Exchange Visitor Sponsorship Program. Visit ECFMG's Web site at www.ecfmg.org/evsp for access to the J-1 Visa Sponsorship Fact Sheet. Its Exchange Visitor Sponsorship Reference Guide provides application materials and important updates.
- U.S. Department of State Exchange Visitor Program (DOS-EVP) at http://exchanges.state.gov/education/jexchanges.
- U.S. Citizenship and Immigration Services at www.uscis.gov.
- U.S. Department of Homeland Security at www.dhs.gov/dhspublic.
- U.S. Embassies and Consulates at http://travel.state.gov/visa/questions_embassy.html.

II Entering a Training Program

Barbara J. Hoekje, PhD, and Marta van Zanten, MEd

Communication Skills   71

Language and Culture   71

Communication in Clinical Settings   72

Medicalese   73

Communicating with Patients   73

- *The Doctor-Patient Relationship and the Diagnostic Interview*   74

- *Forms of Address*   74

Communication with Other Members of the Health Care Team   75

- *Talking about Patients*   76

Writing in Clinical Settings   76

Communication in Educational Settings   76

Communication in Social Settings   77

Making Small-Talk   77

Getting the Floor and Interrupting   78

Nonverbal Communication   78

Back-Channel Cues   79

Personal Space   79

Eye Contact   79

Gestures   80

Touch   80

First Impressions   81

- *Handshakes and Introductions*   81

- *Dress and Body Smells*   81

Assessment of Communication and English Proficiency Skills in a Medical Environment — 82

Spoken English Proficiency Requirement — 82

Communication and Interpersonal Skills Requirement — 83

Self-Assessment of English Proficiency Skills — 83

Improving Communication Skills — 84

World Varieties of English — 85

Identifying Problems and Accessing Resources — 85

Ensuring Comprehension and Learning to Listen — 86

Expanding Repertoires and Skills: Language and Cultural Diversity — 86

Summary — 87

Communication Skills

Communicating effectively as a doctor involves mastery of many forms of language, from the more formal style of the workplace to informal conversation with co-workers and peers. Doctors use language to interview patients to get the information they need for diagnostic purposes and to establish the rapport that will facilitate treatment. Good communication skills increase the effectiveness of clinical performance through increased accuracy of information elicited from the patient and increased efficiency in getting the information. More effective communication skills result in improved satisfaction for doctor and patient, a better therapeutic relationship between them, increased patient compliance and efficiency of care, and better health outcomes for the patient.

Physicians who are not fully comfortable with the English language may have difficulty interviewing patients and understanding their narratives and concerns and may also have trouble interacting with their patients' family members and other medical staff. In addition, many malpractice claims have been shown to be the result of a physician's poor communication skills and a lack of understanding between the doctor and patient.

The Accreditation Council for Graduate Medical Education (ACGME) now includes interpersonal and communication skills "that result in effective information exchange and teaming with patients, their families, and other health professionals" as one of its six core competencies for physician education.

Due to workforce needs, training opportunities, and the overall globalization of medicine, many physicians who do not speak English as their first language choose to practice medicine in English-speaking countries such as the United States. Internationally trained physicians are not evenly distributed across the United States. Therefore, depending on where an international medical graduate (IMG) chooses to practice, patients and other health care team individuals may or may not be accustomed to interacting with someone who is from another culture or who does not speak English as his or her first language.

This chapter reviews the foundations of effective communication in the medical workplace and academic and social settings, beginning with some of the general features of language use in the United States. Issues of non-verbal behaviors and listening skills are also addressed because they are a crucial part of effective communication. Because IMGs seeking to enter GME in the United States are obligated to demonstrate appropriate English language skills as part of certification exams, information is provided regarding official language requirements. The chapter ends with suggestions and resources for addressing and improving communication skills.

LANGUAGE AND CULTURE

Language expresses cultural values in both its forms and uses. While much diversity exists in the United States, interpersonal interactions are generally friendly, direct, and non-hierarchical. In public, people greet each other with cheerful expressions of interest ("Hi! How are you?" "What's up?") and leave with similar expressions ("Have a good weekend!" "See you later!"). Newcomers to the United States sometimes find these friendly greetings to be a misleading sign of true friendship rather than simply a verbal style of interaction. Friendly greetings express the positive outlook and cheerful and pragmatic perspective that is a U.S. cultural value. Directness means speaking one's own intentions, interests, and point of view. In a highly individualistic society like the United

States, speakers are expected to present themselves and their interests straightforwardly rather than waiting for others to anticipate or try to figure them out. Excessive modesty is not seen as a value, although overestimation of one's talents or contributions (bragging) is also not appreciated. Taking someone "at their word" or "at face value" reflects the pragmatic expectation that self-representation should be honest and forthright. IMGs who are used to more modest ways of speaking may need to practice identifying their strengths and wishes in a direct manner in interviewing and other settings.

People who are aggressive in advocating for themselves or family members in health care or other situations may just be following the adage, "The squeaky wheel gets the grease," an expression which acknowledges that those who speak loudest usually get the most attention. In problem areas between doctors and patients, worried patients may press doctors overly aggressively. Yet physicians may not be aware of the anxiety of the silent patient who does not speak up about these and other significant issues.

In cases of conflict, individuals are expected to first try to resolve matters directly by having a talk to "hash things out" because "there are two sides to every story." A person who speaks badly about another person to a third party is seen as "talking behind the back" of the other person and being "two-faced." Many resources exist about how to raise and resolve interpersonal issues of conflict well. The American Medical Association (AMA) online resource *Virtual Mentor* (August 2005 issue) has sample scripts for dealing with difficult conversations in the health care context; these are available at http://virtualmentor.ama-assn.org/2005/08/toc-0508.html.

If residents are dissatisfied with any aspect of their program, they should bring the issue to the administrative staff with responsibility for the issue. Most often that will be the program director. Going to a higher level, such as bringing a complaint or a concern to the Graduate Medical Education dean's office is considered "going over the head" of the program director, who is likely to feel disrespected. Only in extreme cases should this be done, not as routine practice.

In the United States, language expresses a non-hierarchical perspective that is a cultural value. Starting from the pronoun *you*, which is used to address both the President of the United States as well as the youngest child, English is a language with fewer forms of distinction between formal and informal and between high status and low status than many other languages. IMGs may be used to more deference to authority in their home countries than is expressed in the United States, including unquestioning acceptance of what they say as physicians. In the United States, doctors are frequently questioned or even argued with by patients. This may be a sign of an increasing sense of consumer rights that has spread into the health care arena and from patient empowerment through Internet chat groups. Television shows such as ER and *House* also create an image of hospital medicine that can affect the way patients talk with their doctors in real life or their expectations of treatment. Doctors are expected to show patients mutual respect in use of names (using titles in addressing their patients, at least initially) and to modify their own language so that patients understand and feel comfortable in speaking with them. In all cases, doctors are held to professional standards of conduct in communication no matter what the verbal behaviors of their patients.

Communication in Clinical Settings

When a new resident steps into a hospital or other health care setting, he or she enters a community where work is done according to a particular set of rules, many of which are unspoken and unwritten. Many riveting narratives and anthropological treatises have been written about the process of becoming acculturated to this new environment by medical students and residents and are listed in this chapter's references. These stories have noted some of the unique ways of using language that occur within the medical profession and hospital place of practice. One stereotype of the way doctors communicate is their use of a form of language known as *medicalese*.

MEDICALESE

Medicalese is a trade jargon used by medical personnel who typically work closely with each other over time and develop a shorthand way of talking about their work that includes many abbreviations, acronyms, slang expressions, and technical vocabulary. Some of these terms are common across medical settings, and some are restricted to a particular workplace. Some examples are acronyms such as "CHF" for congestive heart failure, word clippings such as "crit" for hemocrit, and slang such as "blow" for destroying a vein while inserting an IV. Studies of doctors' communications show the importance of avoiding medicalese in their conversations with patients. Use of specialized vocabulary is especially problematic when the word has a meaning in more common language as well (e.g., *depression*, *eating disorder*). Somewhat in contrast to this, in the United States drugs are often referred to by their brand name (e.g., Tylenol) rather than by their chemical composition (e.g., acetaminophen), even in communications with other members of the health care team. Doctors need to find the balance between technical terminology and more commonly used terms in their communications, keeping in mind the twin goals of accuracy and comprehensibility.

COMMUNICATING WITH PATIENTS

Beyond the use of technical language, communicating effectively with patients presents a number of other challenges, including the fact that patients may be sick, in pain, and on medication; they may speak local nonstandard varieties of English or other languages; they may be very old and have hearing loss or difficulty with speech. Reticent or shy patients may use euphemistic or vague terms (e.g., "thingy") in discussing sensitive matters. Young children present another set of communication issues. Many words relating to bodily functions and activities have a child version different from the adult version (e.g., "go potty" "belly button, "tummy ache") that IMGs might not be familiar with. Working with children and adolescents also requires communication skills in providing information and reassurance to parents. These and other aspects can make it challenging for new residents to communicate effectively, especially in the early phases of their work in a new patient setting.

Since the doctor-patient relationship is so central to good health care delivery, training should be given to develop and assess doctors' communication skills and other skills related to building this relationship. Research confirms the importance of doctor communication in patient satisfaction. Primary care doctors who spend more time with their patients (even just a few more minutes) and who use such communication behaviors to check understanding, ask opinions and encourage talk, humor, and appropriate language are significantly less likely to be sued in malpractice suits than doctors who do not.

It is also important that a doctor maintain a balance in expression of attitude when communicating with patients. Most patients prefer that the doctor convey therapeutic confidence when communicating. In other words, the doctor should engender a feeling that he or she can help the patient, without being too overconfident or making unrealistic promises. If the doctor is unsure of something, it is appropriate to inform the patient of the uncertainty and reassure the patient that he or she will find the answer.

The Doctor-Patient Relationship and the Diagnostic Interview

Much of the research on doctor-patient communication has focused on the diagnostic interview, where the doctor elicits information from the patient to help make a diagnosis. While much of the earlier research focused on specific behaviors of the physician, newer research puts more emphasis on the effect of the doctor's language on the patient and vice versa. The doctor's questions can help the patient understand his or her thinking, and the patient's information can help inform the doctor. It is important that the doctor listen to the patient's story of his or her illness rather than approaching the patient with a pre-conceived idea.

Doctors' questioning techniques can help or hinder the patient's description of his or her illness. In the most effective interview, the doctor allows the patient more room in telling his or her narrative even when information may seem initially irrelevant rather than maintaining a tight structure of questioning. Allowing patients time to tell the story of why they have come to the doctor in their own words is very important. In fact, both open-ended and close-ended questions can be useful in patient interviews. One model of the interview can be seen as consisting of a sequence of five stages structured by the doctor:

1. *Initiating the session*—Establish initial rapport and identify the reason(s) for the consultation.
2. *Gathering information*—Explore the patient's problems.
3. *Physical examination*—Advise patient of maneuvers before doing them, especially if painful or sensitive; respect patient's modesty and comfort during examination.
4. *Explanation and planning*—Provide the correct amount and type of information; aid accurate recall and understanding; achieve a shared understanding incorporating the patient's perspective; use shared decision making to plan.
5. *Closing the session*—Plan for the future and provide appropriate closure.

Each of these tasks has a series of communication moves associated with them. The full structure of this interview framework is available online at www.gp-training.net/training/theory/calgary/calgary.pdf.

Forms of Address

Forms of address are the names used when people speak to each other. A doctor will usually be addressed with title plus last name (e.g., "Dr. Liu"). In recent years, there has been more awareness about the importance of doctors using reciprocal naming patterns with patients—that is, using a title plus last name (e.g., "Mr. Singh") to mitigate concerns of disrespect or inequality. Women may be addressed with the title "Ms" (pronounced "Mizz") plus last name if their marital status is not known or "Mrs." (Missus) for married women or "Miss" for unmarried women. Children may be addressed by their first name.

Patients may invite their doctors to call them by their first name ("Call me Sandy"), but physicians should not initiate first naming on their own or ask patient permission to do so. Should doctors invite patients to address them by first name? There is no hard-and-fast rule; however, doctors who allow first naming should realize that there is a consequence to this in terms of the establishment of authority. For example, an Asian female doctor in a pediatric service who allowed first naming along with the rest of the health care team found herself frequently mistaken for a nurse.

In the residency training program, a supervisor, peer, or co-worker will ideally provide the name they would like to be called by saying, "Please call me Alex" for example, but this does not always occur. It will be helpful for IMGs to also provide the name they would like to be called, especially if they have helpful nicknames or difficult names that bear repeating. Clarifying expectations around names will avoid the use of the no-naming strategy, which is when a speaker avoids calling the other person by name because of discomfort or insecurity about the appropriate choice. In the absence of clarification, it is probably best to follow the general practices of peers in the case of terms of address with supervisors and co-workers.

Finally, it is worth noting that what English speakers call first and last names do not always correspond to given and surname names. Chinese is one language where surnames are the first of the two names, so that a person named "Hu Lin" has a surname of "Hu" and a given name of "Lin." In English, this person may ask to be called "Lin" or "Hu" and may even switch the order around to conform to English standards, which may confuse the situation when submitting forms for official purposes. Spanish names are another case where a person may have three names such as "Carlos Hernandez Piedra." In this case, the first of the two family names will often, but not always, serve as his formal "last" name for English database purposes (Box 5-1).

☑ BOX 5-1   **Best Practices in Talking with Patients**

- Avoid medicalese (abbreviations, acronyms, specialized vocabulary).
- Use open-ended questions and allow patient to narrate the story in his or her own words.
- Check comprehension on both sides through comprehension checks, restatement, and written support.
- Use title plus last name with adults until invited to do otherwise.
- With pediatric patients, remember the dual requirements of communication (children and parents).

COMMUNICATION WITH OTHER MEMBERS OF THE HEALTH CARE TEAM

The team approach is an area that has been identified as a core feature of U.S. health care culture. Good communication helps to establish and build rapport and good working relationships with other members of the health care team. Appropriate protocols of communication include resolving any issues of treatment outside of the patient's presence. The AMA *Virtual Mentor* (http://virtualmentor.ama-assn.org/2005/08/toc-0508.html) gives a vignette where a nurse disagrees with a doctor about the way a problem has been handled. This situation may be unthinkable in other countries where the nurse's role is much more limited in scope. As the commentator notes, in the United States nurses have independent professional accountability to the patient's welfare and the responsible practice of medicine. The American Association of Colleges of Nursing (AACN) describes the role of the nurse as follows:

> *Nurses are providers of care. In this role, nurses are patients' advocates and educators. Historically, the nursing role has emphasized partnership with patients—whether individuals, families, groups, or communities—in order to foster and support active participation in determining health care decisions. Patient advocacy is, and will continue to be, a hallmark of the professional nursing role, and requires that nurses deliver high quality care, evaluate care outcomes, and provide leadership in improving care. (p. 4)*

Doctors who come from traditions where the scope of nursing is much more limited should educate themselves about the scope of responsibility held by U.S. nurses and seek best practices in effective communication with nurses and other members of the health care team.

Talking about Patients

As many signs posted in the hospital will remind the health care team, doctors must take care not to discuss patients in public areas. In addition, patients should not be referred to by their disease, physical characteristics, room numbers or other terms that depersonalize or demean the patient. Such terminology arises out of the pressure of the work environment, socialization practices that at times emphasize the doctors at the expense of the patients, and natural processes of workplace communication where people who work consistently together over time develop shorthand terminology and insider slang. Although the use of disrespectful language has been part of medical culture for some time, it has no place in the professional practice of medicine and should be interrupted and repaired. See the American Medical Association's online journal *Virtual Mentor* (special issue on communication) for a sample script for repairing a potential break in trust between a patient's family and the health care team due to a doctor's use of a derogatory term for a comatose patient.

WRITING IN CLINICAL SETTINGS

Documentation in the medical record warrants special consideration and is extensively addressed in Chapter 7. However, a few points may be made with respect to issues particularly relevant to IMGs. Certain words or phrases that an IMG may be accustomed to writing in patient records in their home countries may not be commonly used in the United States. While technically not incorrect, these phrases may cause confusion to other members of the health care team who are unaware of their meaning. For example, it is appropriate in some international training environments to use fractions to specify duration of an illness or condition, such as 2/52 to indicate two weeks, or 3/24 to indicate three hours. That use of duration of time fractions is not common in the United States and could pose problems of interpretation by those who read the patient record. Other examples of non-standard written English in patient records include the use of the word "refers" in place of "has" or "indicates" (e.g., "He refers no pain"), the use of "nil" when indicating that something is not applicable or non-contributory, and the use of value-laden terms such as "fornicate" in place of the more neutral "sexually active".

Communication in Educational Settings

Communication in the academic portion of graduate medical education includes participation in lecture and discussion settings, orientations, conferences, and rounds. In general, the American classroom is an interactive and participatory setting where students are expected to ask questions, make comments, contribute new perspectives, and draw their own conclusions about information. International residents who come from traditions where lecturers give information that is to be learned as a body of received information may find it difficult to adjust to the U.S. academic expectations. However, it is important that they do so, as remaining quiet in the classroom or on rounds may be judged as passivity or lack of preparation. The prepared student who brings his or her own relevant experience and knowledge to the discussion at hand will be judged more active and involved in learning. At the same time, dominating the discussion is not appreciated or valued by either the faculty or other students in the course. Students who come from different traditions may need to watch other effective contributors for model behavior in the initial period. It is important to learn how to answer questions put to the class as a whole rather than to specific students by name, because this method is a common questioning technique in U.S. classrooms.

Information in presentations and other prepared talks should be original, clear, brief, and deductive. A prepared talk should not begin with an apology, especially not one that begs the audience's forgiveness for the speaker's lack of preparation. In some other countries, this ritual apology is an expected part of the speech, but in the United States it is likely to be taken at face value and undermine the speaker's credibility.

Residents will also be expected to submit papers as part of coursework as well as eventually contribute to medical journals and other publications. Learning to write well about medicine for publication in various professional or academic journals also takes time and attention, but it is a skill that can be learned. Many good guides are available (see References).

Plagiarism, or academic dishonesty, is a major concern in higher education and the intellectual tradition generally. Under no circumstances can other people's ideas be used without proper attribution. As medical residents become educated to join the professional medical community both in the United States and through international conferences, they must learn proper protocol for citing other sources. Some problems in proper attribution arise unintentionally through insufficient care in note-taking or lack of understanding of the rules of attribution. But the consequences of plagiarism can be swift and severe, and the judgment against the plagiarizer is unequivocal. Anyone who is unclear about norms in this area should seek help from a reference librarian or academic advisor. The American Medical Association's *Manual of Style* (see References) provides useful information on this and many other topics.

Communication in Social Settings

Communication in social settings can present challenges for speakers who have learned and used English mostly in professional or academic contexts. Conversational language is characterized by fast and elided speech and idiomatic and slang expressions. Topics of conversation move quickly and tend to be based on local cultural knowledge and humor rather than on an academic or professional knowledge base.

MAKING SMALL-TALK

In a society so large and diverse, discussions of religion and politics in the United States can often expose major differences in belief and lead to serious argument. These kinds of discussions are usually avoided in casual social conversation. *Small-talk* is the term for social interaction with language that is intended primarily to show friendly intent without risking serious values conflict. Topics for small talk include the weather, sports, movies, shopping, and other common activities. Weather is an enduring topic stemming from the U.S. farming heritage as well as from its intrinsic changeability. Sports are of enormous interest, especially American football, basketball, and baseball. IMGs and all those relocating to a new place who develop loyalty to the local teams and players will find an open door to conversations with their patients, other members of the health care team, and neighbors. Sports have influenced American English, and there are many sports metaphors in everyday use (Box 5-2).

☑ **BOX 5-2   Some Sports Metaphors in Everyday Use**

From Baseball
1. *To step up to the plate*: To take responsibility
2. *To bat a thousand*: To be consistently correct or a winner, or, used ironically, to be consistently wrong or a loser
3. *Three strikes and you're out*: After three failed attempts, it is someone else's turn to attempt the task at hand
4. *To be out in left field*: To be out of touch or not in the normal range of ideas, common sense, etc.
5. *To come out of left field*: To unexpectedly appear without warning or context
6. *To be off base*; To be wrong, to be out of line
7. *To pinch hit*: To stand in for, or take the place of, someone else
8. *Right off the bat*: Immediately, directly

From Basketball
1. *To be a slam dunk*: To be an easily accomplished goal

From Football
1. *To take the ball and run with it*: To take action
2. *To do an end run*: To circumvent
3. *To tackle a problem*: To confront it directly

GETTING THE FLOOR AND INTERRUPTING

Conversation in the United States generally consists of continually overlapping lines of talk, incomplete sentences, and pauses, restarts, rephrasing, and repetitions. Talk is organized differently in different cultures, with different norms about how speakers get and keep the floor. Learning how to get into the conversation takes skill and understanding of these rules because turns of talk go back and forth very quickly. Both the current speaker and the one who wants to speak send signals about their intention to change turns. The current speaker signals his or her end of turn through repetition of the main point, use of discourse markers (e.g., "So...") and filler words, and falling intonation and slowing speech. The one who wants to speak cannot wait until the first speaker is completely finished to start talking. Instead, he or she must make slight forward body movement and small sounds or movements that signal his or her intent. Usually the turn transfer between speakers happens so quickly and smoothly that one person begins talking before the other has ended. A speaker who does not know how to manage this transition will end up interrupting inappropriately. Time, practice, and attention to these practices will help.

Nonverbal Communication

Communication includes both verbal (language) and nonverbal aspects. Nonverbal communication includes personal space, eye contact, gestures, body movements, and touch. Nonverbal communication sends powerful messages that often operate underneath the speakers' awareness. The physical gestures and movements of two people in conversation can be seen as culturally patterned interaction, in which the actions of one are intricately coordinated to the actions of the other, from eye contact to head movement to hand movement. In cases when both speakers are operating with the same set of cultural patterns, the speakers feel that they are "in sync"—and they literally are. However, when operating within two different systems, speakers may feel that they don't see "eye to eye" with another speaker. They may also come to different conclusions about the meaning of a nonverbal action. Because so much meaning is communicated nonverbally, IMGs must become aware of potential areas for conflict in their nonverbal actions. IMGs should seek feedback on situations where intent was misunderstood, because these situations may result from cross-cultural behaviors and unintentional messages.

BACK-CHANNEL CUES

Back-channel cues is a term that refers to the many forms of feedback that a listener gives to a speaker while he or she is talking to signal attention and interest. Back-channel cues include small head nods, eye contact, small sounds ("Hmm...", "Oh!", etc.) and facial expressions. Some listeners are more expressive than others, but generally American English speakers give many back-channel cues in conversation. Not all cultures give back-channel cues to the extent or in the same way as American English speakers. The up-and-down head nod and raised eyebrows used by Greek speakers signals "no" rather than "yes" for example, and Asian Indian speakers have a sideways nod to acknowledge "yes" that can look like "no" to Americans. Some speakers from other cultures give fewer back-channel cues in speaking and can seem distant, inattentive, or nonresponsive in conversation. Doctors need to use back-channel cues when interviewing patients or listening to others to signal attention and interest, especially when they are not able to use eye contact (e.g., on the telephone).

PERSONAL SPACE

"Personal space" refers to the area around the self in which people in a culture feel comfortable. The anthropologist Edward Hall categorized the distance middle-class Americans usually keep between each other as having four ranges: intimate, personal, social, and public. Personal distance in the United States ranges from arm's length between people to easy touching distance (from about 4 to 1.5 feet), whereas intimate space is closer and involves sensory perception of body heat, body smells, and visual distortion. The miscommunication that can occur when people with different personal space boundaries interact can be powerful and upsetting. If a person with one set of boundaries moves into the intimate space of another without realizing it, the second person might feel that the first has invaded his or her space. The first person may find himself or herself characterized as personally aggressive or making sexual advances. In the opposite case, a speaker who stands too far away might be characterized as distant, cold, standoffish, or somehow strange. Doctors must enter intimate space when they are in the clinical setting doing physical examination or performing procedures, but in other settings this will make others uncomfortable and is likely to be misinterpreted.

EYE CONTACT

Eye contact refers to the degree to which two speakers look each other in the eye when talking. It is common in the United States to have much eye contact between speakers, with the listener looking at the speaker and the speaker regularly glancing at the listener. This occurs in nearly all situations, from the classroom to one-on-one talk. When a speaker does not look at the listener, he or she is likely to be judged as shifty or untrustworthy. A listener who does not maintain eye contact with the speaker may be judged inattentive or bored. During physical examinations such as gynecological exams, visual boundaries may be established that separate the doctor's visual gaze from that of the patient. But in other situations such as interviewing, doctors should use eye contact to help establish rapport. This can be especially challenging when the doctor wishes to take notes during history taking, as it is necessary to maintain a reasonable amount of eye contact with the patient while simultaneously writing. In this situation it is appropriate for a doctor to first ask a patient, "Is it OK if I take notes while we talk? Please know that I am listening to you while I write", or "I'm still listening, I'm just taking a few notes while you speak so I don't miss anything". Informing a patient of note taking allows the patient to expect less eye contact from the doctor than would generally be considered appropriate in other one-on-one communication settings.

GESTURES

Gestures are the movements of the hands, head, and body as part of the communication stream during talk or as representative sign. While many facial expressions are common across human cultures, misinterpretation may still occur when cultural meaning is attached to these expressions (e.g., the smile that expresses embarrassment rather than humor). Gestures are also culturally determined and can cause miscommunication. For example, the gestures for "Come here" and "Go away" are different in different countries, and IMGs should pay close attention to the way these are done in the United States to be sure their own gestures correspond.

The use of the middle finger in almost any outstretched position is taboo in the United States because of the strong insulting connotations of "giving the finger" to someone. However, in some other countries people use the middle finger as a pointing finger or as a non-significant gesture in say, pushing up one's glasses. The consequences of using the middle finger unintentionally are so powerful that anyone doing this should be privately advised.

TOUCH

While a reassuring touch can be a most welcome sign of encouragement or support, unwelcome touch is invasive. For a doctor, whose touch is a direct source of diagnostic information, touch has professional implications as well as interpersonal meaning. In general, touch is quite limited in U.S. professional and social circles except among intimates (parents and children, lovers, caregivers) and in some sports. In public, friends do not hold hands or link arms as they do in many countries in Asia or Latin America. Male friends do not stand with their arms over each others' shoulders as they do in Arab and some other countries. Adult patients who live alone or who are not in an intimate relationship may have little occasion to be touched outside of clinical or caregiver settings. The emphasis on sexual harassment in the workplace is such that health care professionals—especially those in positions of authority such as teachers or team leaders—should be extremely cautious about touching anyone, even as a gesture of support. In fact, outside the clinical setting, touching in the workplace is virtually a taboo.

The actual clinical encounter is a unique situation with respect to touch. Even in the absence of belief in any healing power of "laying on of hands," physicians have noted that many patients feel reassured by their applying a stethoscope to the chest or heart or by palpating the abdomen, even when these maneuvers are not clearly indicated based on the patient's complaint.

FIRST IMPRESSIONS

Handshakes and Introductions

In most professional settings in the United States, two people will shake hands the first time they meet. The accomplishment of the handshake in introductions, along with a smile, eye contact and the mutual "How do you do?" is an intricate and mutually accomplished sequence and can set the tone for the ongoing relationship. IMGs who come from cultures that do not use handshakes to greet and who are uncomfortable with this routine should be given many opportunities to watch, practice, and learn this routine as it is a key social practice. It is also worth noting that the use of the handshake can differ by gender. Depending on age, custom, and region, some women do not as readily shake hands as men do. Men and women should be aware of this. If the woman you are meeting makes no movement to extend her hand, simply say the greeting without the handshake.

All doctors meeting patients for the first time or after an extended time should introduce themselves and give their role on the health care team. Although this seems obvious, it is omitted surprisingly often. IMGs should be careful to give their name slowly, spelling it or pointing to the nametag where it is written for extra visual support so that patients can more easily remember it. Saying the name in English phonology may make it easier for patients to access and remember it as well. Confirming the patient's name and preferred form of address should be done in all cases, beginning first by addressing the patient by title and full name—for example, "Ms Evelyn Wang."

Dress and Body Smells

Norms of appropriate dress in a society are learned through the many occasions of professional and social life. Relative to many countries where dress is more formal and people tend to have fewer but often more elegant clothes, Americans wear a greater number of outfits. Wearing the same clothes two or more days in a row is culturally frowned upon. People from more conservative countries may be shocked at U.S. fashion styles, especially for women and young people, who may be tattooed and pierced in numerous places. Doctors should be aware that there is not necessarily a connection between the wearer's clothing style and tattoos and his or her morals or beliefs. In some situations it may be appropriate for the physician in the clinical setting to explore the meaning of clothing, tattoos, and piercing for the wearer.

In the United States, norms around body odors are that most of the body's natural smells are masked. While all doctors must learn specific protocols about hygiene and cleanliness, newcomers to the United States may face more issues in this area due to changes in climate, diet, frequency of laundering clothes, showering, and customs about shaving armpits and wearing deodorant. Many people in the United States wash their hair every day, for example, and many women shave their legs and underarms.

Dress, body smells, eye contact and smiles, and the initial handshake all contribute to the first impression that the doctor makes to his or her patients or fellow health professionals. Workshops or private advice given to the IMG may be useful for any doctor with very different norms in this area. A list of taboos on this and other topics is given in Box 5-3.

☑ BOX 5-3   **Taboo Verbal and Nonverbal Behaviors in U.S. Professional Contexts**

- Gesturing, pointing, etc., with the middle finger
- Strong, unpleasant natural body smells including breath
- Touching others except in highly appropriate settings
- Jokes or derogatory statements that make reference to sexual, ethnic, religious, or racial identity

---

Assessment of Communication and English Proficiency Skills in a Medical Environment

IMGs training in residency programs in the United States come from virtually every country in the world, and approximately three quarters do not speak English as a first language. To ensure that these doctors can communicate effectively, performance-based evaluations have been widely used to assess a physician's ability to interact with patients in a simulated clinical environment. The format of a simulated medical assessment is often referred to as an objective structured clinical examination (OSCE). In an OSCE, physician examinees rotate through a series of stations, encountering a different standardized, or simulated, patient (SP) in each room. SPs are persons who realistically portray patients with physical or psychological clinical complaints, such as depression, recurring headaches, and abdominal pain. SPs are trained in the role of a particular patient, expressing in every encounter the same complaint, past medical history, social history, response to physical exam maneuvers, etc. In most OSCEs, physician examinees are aware that the SPs are actors simulating their complaints, not real patients. Nevertheless, examinees are instructed to interact with the SPs as they would with actual patients, questioning the patients about their illnesses, performing physical exams, counseling patients on risky behaviors, and providing SPs with information about possible diagnosis and follow-up plans.

Depending on the purpose of the exercise, OSCEs vary in length and administration format. In most OSCEs modeled on a first-time visit, ambulatory care design, examinees are given approximately 15 minutes to interview and examine each patient. Immediately following each encounter, SPs document the clinical skills of the examinees, usually by completing a case-specific checklist indicating which history items were asked and which physical exam maneuvers were performed correctly according to predetermined protocols. In addition, SPs often evaluate the communication and interpersonal skills of the physicians using either checklists or rating scales. A measure of the spoken language skills of non-native English speaking physicians who will be entering the workforce in an English speaking country is an important aspect of ensuring physician competency, and some OSCEs incorporate an evaluation of the physician examinees' spoken language proficiency. If the purpose of the OSCE is formative, following the encounter the SP or a faculty observer will provide the doctor with feedback on his or her performance. They discuss strengths and weaknesses and offer advice on how the doctor can improve clinical skills and communication with patients.

SPOKEN ENGLISH PROFICIENCY REQUIREMENT

IMGs who wish to pursue GME training in the United States must be certified by the Educational Commission for Foreign Medical Graduates (ECFMG). From July 1998 until

June 2004, requirements for ECFMG certification included an acceptable score on the Test of English as a Foreign Language (TOEFL) and passing status on the Clinical Skills Assessment (CSA). The CSA was an OSCE used to ensure that IMGs could demonstrate clinical skills at a level comparable to United States medical graduates (USMGs). Since May 2004, the TOEFL requirement has been eliminated, and the CSA has been replaced by the USMLE Step 2 clinical skills (CS) exam, which is now a requirement for both U.S. medical graduates (USMGs) and IMGs. The CS examination also contains a measure of the physician's spoken English proficiency. Therefore all medical school graduates, regardless of where they went to medical school, seeking to enter into an accredited residency training program in the United States, are now required to demonstrate appropriate clinical and communication skills.

In the currently required CS spoken English proficiency assessment, SPs are trained to judge the overall effectiveness of the physician's communication skills. They evaluate the potential occurrences of breakdowns in communication due to the physician's lack of language skills, such as incorrect, confusing word choices or incomprehensible pronunciation. Therefore the English proficiency assessment is not simply whether or not the doctor spoke with a foreign accent. Although physicians are not required to speak like a native speaker of American English, they are expected to be able to maintain a threshold of language skills necessary to effectively communicate with patients.

COMMUNICATION AND INTERPERSONAL SKILLS REQUIREMENT

As part of the CS exam, SPs also evaluate the interpersonal skills of the examinees. These competencies are assessed along three dimensions; information gathering, information sharing and professional manner and rapport. The rating scales incorporate aspects of doctor-patient communication that are not necessarily directly related to language proficiency, such as maintaining appropriate eye contact and conducting a physical exam respectful of the patient's modesty and comfort. Results of IMG performance on the CS reveal that an internationally-trained physician's skills on subcomponents of the exam are moderated by his or her English proficiency. Physicians with language proficiency below a certain threshold have additional difficulty with other components of the exam. For example, physicians who scored poorly on the measure of English proficiency also were likely to exhibit lower level bedside manner skills, such as their ability to establish rapport with patients. These results highlight how English proficiency skills can have a direct impact on many areas of a physician's ability to be an effective health care provider, both in a simulated medical exam setting and in the real world.

SELF-ASSESSMENT OF ENGLISH PROFICIENCY SKILLS

For physicians contemplating coming to the United States who are unsure of their spoken English proficiency skills, it may be useful to first take a screening test. Performance on an assessment of oral language skills will give the physician some indication as to their likelihood of passing the CS exam, before they undertake the expense of registering for the CS and traveling to the US to sit for the exam. Potential test-taker anxiety may also be moderated by first attempting a no-stakes assessment.

There are numerous widely used oral language skills assessments available which are offered in testing centers around the world. The recently revised Test of English as a Foreign Language (TOEFL), administered by the Educational Testing Service (ETS), is a frequently used assessment in North America for evaluating the English skills of non-native speaking individuals seeking to enter educational institutions in the United States or for certification and licensure of certain occupations. The TOEFL measures the ability of nonnative speakers of English to use and understand English as it is spoken, written, and heard in college and university settings. The TOEFL Internet-based test (iBT) measures integrated communication competency in all four language areas: reading, listening, writing, and speaking. The TOEFL versions that were previously required for ECFMG certification are no longer being offered by ETS. Therefore, while the TOEFL does not specifically measure English proficiency in a medical environment, and direct comparisons between scores received on the TOEFL exam and potential performance on the CS cannot be made, the TOEFL will certainly give someone unsure of his or her English ability a reasonable idea of level of performance. Currently the minimum TOEFL spoken component score required for non-native English-speaking individuals seeking certification in other health care fields is 26. Physicians who receive a score of 26 or higher on the spoken component of the TOEFL can expect to do reasonably well on the Spoken English Proficiency component of the CS.

The Test of English for International Communication (TOEIC), also administered by ETS, is a test of English proficiency that has been used as a standard for establishing business English writing skills and spoken English proficiency. Institutions, companies, and government agencies worldwide use TOEIC as a standard for establishing English proficiency in potential employees. Information on both the TOEFL and the TOEIC tests can be found on the ETS Web site (http://www.ets.org).

The Cambridge International English Language Testing Service (IELTS) test is an English language proficiency test designed for academic and professional English language assessment. It tests speaking, listening, reading, and writing and reports scores in nine general bands. Numerous levels of exams are offered, from an assessment of basic language skills to very advanced. Testing centers are located throughout the world, including the United States. For more information, visit www.ielts.org.

Improving Communication Skills

In response to the many studies accumulating research on the value of good communication in medicine and the many problems identified in the communication area, teaching and assessing communication skills is now a common part of medical training through use of standardized patients (SP) and other pedagogy (www.virtualmentor.org). Even for doctors who passed the spoken English proficiency component of the CS exam, it is important to remember that this assessment is of minimum competency, and successful communication in the U.S. health care environment may require a higher ability level. Communication can be improved through practice, especially in the difficult areas for discussion that can occur with both patients and non-patients. While there are best practices in communication, there is rarely one right answer, as communication is intricately tied to the specific context and people communicating. There is value in studying model scripts for such conversations and considering the ramifications of choosing one or another response. *Virtual Mentor* (Volume 7, Number 8, August 2005) gives seven vignettes of difficult conversations along with expert commentary. These vignettes include physician-to-patient communication (Vignette 1) in disclosing error, colleague-to-colleague communication (Vignette 3) in confronting a colleague about poor performance, physician-to-nurse communication (Vignette 4) about lack of respect, resident-to-student communication (Vignette 7) about giving feedback on performance, and others.

For some IMGs, the various language choices they may wish to use in a speech situation can merit preparation ahead of time. This can include time and practice with scripts or modeling language and behaviors from others who are recognized as excellent communicators in the department. Finding opportunities to get feedback on communication skills is extremely important for IMGs, both in initial stages of practice and often again at the end of residency as they prepare for independent practice with a different clientele and setting.

WORLD VARIETIES OF ENGLISH

Some of the discussion in this chapter may be more applicable to those who have learned English as a subsequent language to their first language. Yet speakers of other world varieties of English as a mother tongue may also face communication difficulties as they take up practice in U.S. health care contexts. The world varieties of English occur in places such as India and Nigeria where there has been long-term institutional incorporation of English into the educational and other institutions of society. In these different Englishes, words mean different things; for example, "fag", "knock up" and "rubber" all have sexual connotations in American English but not necessarily in other varieties. Other terms, such as "return trip" (round trip) and "occupied" (phone is busy), can also cause confusion.

Speakers of other-world Englishes may also come from places where more formality is expected. Use of the direct address "ma'am", for example, is respectful in India but is not generally used in the United Sates outside of the South. Other traditions in the English-speaking world differ. In Great Britain, for example, going out after work with your attending physician may lead to a completely different level of formality, including different naming patterns, whereas a formality shift to that extent is less likely in the United States.

Speakers of other-world varieties of English have different patterns of stress and intonation that can greatly influence the way that a sentence is interpreted. For example, a high pitch fall may sound imperious or condescending, whereas a final intonational rise may sound uncertain and weak. The English of other-world varieties when spoken rapidly with a different stress and intonation contour and accompanied by different head and eye movements can be incomprehensible to those who are only familiar with an American accent. Speakers of other-world varieties of English need to be particularly attuned to potential miscommunication, especially in initial stages.

IDENTIFYING PROBLEMS AND ACCESSING RESOURCES

As may be evident from the discussion above, communication can break down between doctors and their patients or co-workers in any one of a variety of ways: from the actual code itself—the comprehensibility of the form of the language—to miscommunication due to word choice and ways of speaking in both medical and everyday language. Fortunately there are ways that residents can improve their communication skills. Sometimes it is a simple matter of training residents in appropriate genre and form (e.g., tightening up presentations to conform to time and organization expectations). There may also be a need for residents to become more familiar with the language of the patient community, including local and regional varieties of English, and the idioms, slang, and rapid pace of conversational speech.

Some IMGs, even very long-term residents of the United States, can still have significant interference from remnants of their first language or other world varieties of English.

Making these speakers more aware of their language and shaping their speech more toward target language norms can be a painstaking process that can take substantial effort and activity. Speech therapists, ESL experts, and other communication specialists are appropriate referrals for this work. Communication can be improved. Residents often have tuition benefits through their employers that can be used for improvement of communication skills through these referrals. There are a range of curricular options for addressing IMG communication needs in various settings and during the three critical time periods: entry, initial stages of practice, and at the end of residency when establishing an independent practice.

ENSURING COMPREHENSION AND LEARNING TO LISTEN

Good listening skills are an integral part of effective communication. Good listening can refer to the accurate comprehension of information—a necessary first step. Doctors should become vigilant in checking for understanding in communicating with patients through two-way comprehension checks and other means: "Are my patients understanding me? Am I understanding them?" Doctors working with patient populations with regional dialects that are difficult for them to understand may need to consciously provide time for more conversational interaction and listening in the early stages of practice and to always ask for clarification if a word or phrase is not clear. In this way, the doctor can build a lexicon of relevant local terms and pronunciations. Box 5-4 lists tips for checking comprehension.

☑ **BOX 5-4 Tips for Checking and Ensuring Comprehension**

1. Speak slowly when giving key information and watch the patient for nonverbal signs of confusion (puzzled looks, hesitation, etc.).
2. Pause after giving key information and look at the patient. Give the patient a chance to clarify.
3. Ask the patient if he or she has any questions. Show genuine interest and allow waiting time. (Caution! A perfunctory "Do you have any questions?" without waiting time discourages patients.)
4. Ask the patient to repeat or to write down key information.
5. Provide e-mail if appropriate or other resources for follow-up questions.
6. Write down information for patient as appropriate.
7. Ask patients who may have difficulty communicating or understanding to bring a support person with them.

Good listening skills rely on accurate comprehension but go beyond that. When we say of someone, "She's a good listener," we are usually talking about something more. Good listeners provide space for the speaker to speak, but they also provide attention, feedback, and interest. They ask follow-up questions that indicate that they are aware of the trajectory and point of the narrative. They listen for underlying emotion and meaning that might not be present on the surface. *The most interesting people are the most interested people.*

EXPANDING REPERTOIRES AND SKILLS: LANGUAGE AND CULTURAL DIVERSITY

As an additional note about communication, doctors in many patient communities would find a working knowledge of Spanish useful for the many Spanish speakers throughout the United States. On the East Coast, Puerto Rican communities are common; in Florida, Cuban; in the Southwest and West, Mexican. In general, the more culturally and linguistically in tune the doctor can be with the patient and the patient's family, the better. Because of the diversity of many patient communities, it is not possible to know all the patient languages but, over time, learning a few words may be very useful for establishing rapport with the major groups in the patient community. However, notwithstanding the value of establishing rapport by use of some words and terms in a third or fourth language, it is essential that all critical communications, both doctor-to-patient and patient-to-doctor, be verified by a qualified translator.

Most big hospitals provide professional translation services, but if this service is not available problems may arise. Using children or family members is inadvisable because of the censoring of delicate information that might occur either on the part of the patient or the translator. Using anyone who claims to be a speaker of the language is inadvisable because dialect differences are substantial in many languages (Chinese is a good example) and medical symptoms and treatment require expertise in translation. Privacy is also a major concern. For these reasons, a patient who exclusively speaks a language other than English needs special arrangements to communicate with his or her physician. However, it is important for the physician to remember that even when an interpreter is used to communicate with a patient, the actual communication needs to be from doctor to patient, not just doctor to interpreter. Hence, while posing questions, the physician should make efforts to maintain eye contact with and direct facial expressions or gestures to the patient. Similarly, when the interpreter is speaking for the patient, the physician should acknowledge the communication by eye contact and perhaps head nodding to the patient.

For a comprehensive framework for addressing the communication needs of patients from diverse populations who are most at risk for less-than-optimal care, the Ethical Force Program (EFP) of the American Medical Association has engaged in a substantive initiative to improve patient-centered communication. The EFP focuses attention on patient-centered communication as not merely an ethical imperative but as a conduit to better health outcomes. Communication barriers are especially prevalent among vulnerable minority populations, and efforts to improve patient-centered communication may help alleviate racial and ethnic disparities in health care (www.ama-assn.org/ama/pub/category/11929.html).

Because international physicians contribute to workforce diversity, they can often bring insight to cultural diversity and language issues, both areas of focus in the EFP report. The full report, *Improving Communication—Improving Care*, is available at www.ama-assn.org/ama1/pub/upload/mm/369/efimpcomm.pdf. Other resources on working with patients from various cultural groups are available; see, for example, the works by Bigby and by Purnell and Paulanka cited in the Reference section.

Summary

Attention to communication skills is a necessary part of good practice for physicians. International physicians may face additional challenges, especially due to differences in verbal and non-verbal patterns between their style of communication and that of the patient community. Becoming aware of these differences and working through difficulties to develop enhanced communication with patients and other members of the speech community is an endeavor with demonstrated value in patient outcomes and doctor and patient satisfaction.

References

General

Groopman JE. How Doctors Think. Boston: Houghton Mifflin; 2007.

Stone D, Patton B, Heen S. Difficult Conversations: How to Discuss What Matters Most. New York: Viking; 1999.

The Doctoring Experience

Atkinson P. Medical Talk and Medical Work: The Liturgy of the Clinic. London: Sage; 1995.

DasGupta S. Her Own Medicine. New York: Ballantine; 1999.

Konner M. Becoming a Doctor: A Journey of Initiation in Medical School. New York: Viking; 1987.

Medicalese : A Glossary of Medical Terms and Jargon Used in American Medicine. At www.ecfmg.org/acculturation; click on Medicalese link.

Verghese A. My Own Country: A Doctor's Story. New York: Vintage; 1995.

Medical Publishing

Iles RL, Volkland D. Guidebook to Better Medical Writing. Olathe, Kansas: Robert L. Iles; 2003.

JAMA and Archives Journals. AMA Manual of Style, 10 ed. New York: Oxford University Press; 2007.

Taylor RB. The Clinician's Guide to Medical Writing. New York: Springer Science and Business Media; 2005.

Cultural Competency

Bigby J, ed. Cross-Cultural Medicine. Philadelphia: American College of Physicians; 2003.

Purnell LD, Paulanka BJ. Transcultural Health Care: A Culturally Competent Approach. Philadelphia: FA Davis; 1998.

Language

Ong L, De Haes J, Hoose A, Lammes F. Doctor-patient communication: a review of the literature. Soc Sci Med. 1995;40:903–18.

6 American Medical Culture

Gerald P. Whelan, MD

Introduction	90
General American Medical Culture	90
The Missions of American Medical Education	91
Patient Care	91
Medical Education	92
Roles of Residents	92
Physician	92
Student	93
Employee	93
Summary	94

Introduction

There are many definitions of culture, but for our purposes culture refers to the collection of customs, values, priorities, attitudes, beliefs and other factors that are shared by a group of people. Cultural groups range from very large populations existing on the Indian subcontinent, to ethnic groups, to people of one country, or to smaller working groups of people. In reality, every grouping of people working and living together has to some degree their own unique culture, and medicine is no exception. Even more specifically, while there certainly is a culture of American medicine, there are also cultures that characterize subunits of American medicine. Various medical specialties have their own unique cultures, as do different kinds of health care facilities and educational institutions. It would be impossible to define all of these, and there would be exceptions to any such generalizations. So, although we will present some general aspects of the cultures IMGs may encounter in American medicine, it is important to recognize that cultures vary, and the newly arriving IMG should spend some time observing the cultural aspects of the program and institution where he or she is training. The goal is not necessarily to adopt that culture but rather to understand it.

GENERAL AMERICAN MEDICAL CULTURE

Regardless of where or in what specialty an IMG is training, certain cultural elements will be encountered. Perhaps the most obvious on first contact is that American doctors and other health care workers tend to interact fairly informally. Despite position in the hierarchy (see below) all tend to converse fairly freely on a range of topics, often use first names and frequently inject humor into their conversations (see Chapter 5, Language and Communication).

It is often noted that American medicine is considerably less hierarchical than medicine in other countries. While this is true, a hierarchy still exists. Attending physicians are at the top of the hierarchy into which the new IMG resident enters. Many will interact very informally, but this must not be misinterpreted as meaning that they do not expect and deserve the respect of the people they supervise and teach. In addition, each attending has their own unique manner of running the service, rounding and teaching. The best thing for the new IMG to do is observe how their more senior colleagues interact with the attending and emulate that interaction.

Punctuality is highly valued in American medicine. If rounds are to begin at 7:00 a.m., this does not mean 7:30, 7:15 or even 7:05. IMG residents are advised, at least initially, to arrive early for rounds, morning reports, clinics or other scheduled activities. However, although punctuality is valued, the practice of medicine can be unpredictable with respect to time. Patient care, especially any emergencies, always takes precedence over other activities. When unexpected delays cause doctors to be late arriving for patient appointments they should always begin the encounter with an explanation of and an apology for the delay.

Teamwork is a hallmark of American medicine and is addressed in depth elsewhere (see Chapter 8). Relating collegially to other members of the health care team results in more efficient and safer patient care and earns the IMG the respect and support of colleagues. To borrow the saying often used in sports circles, "There is no I in team", meaning that not only is there no letter "I" used in spelling "team", but that there is no place for inflated egos among people who work together as team mates. Teamwork is not only a concept of respect but also requires practical habits like helping another resident who is overwhelmed, being willing to do things that might normally be done by nurses if the situation warrants, or asking colleagues if they want or need help, without waiting to be asked.

Hard work and "pulling your weight", (i.e., doing your share or more of the work that needs to be done) are also highly valued. The term "scut work" has long been used in medicine for tasks that are not necessarily challenging or educationally valuable but simply need to be done, such as drawing blood, obtaining copies of X-rays, taking patients for studies, and changing dressings. Most hospitals recognize that such duties are not the best use of a resident's time and have ancillary staff perform most of them. So, whereas not too long ago in American medicine (and perhaps still in other countries) the first task of the intern, or even the medical student, each morning was to draw blood samples from patients, now a phlebotomy team will do so. Intravenous lines may also be started by phlebotomists or nurses. However, a caution! When nurses or phlebotomists cannot find a vein or get blood, they will ask an intern to do the procedure. Therefore it is imperative to remain proficient in critical skills because emergency situations will arise that require the physician to perform procedures quickly.

The sooner that "scut work" can be completed, the sooner the team can settle down to rounding and teaching; the more help interns give to their team, the more enthusiastic their senior resident will be when teaching them. While it is most appropriate to let staff perform the tasks delegated to them, the intern must be ready to help when the situation warrants.

"Gallows humor" is a term derived from the tendency, even among people heading to the gallows for execution, to find some humor in their situation. It refers to the unique type of humor often manifest among medical staff in America. An example might be the surgeon who wryly observes "All bleeding stops..." The need for gallows humor arises from the stress of working in an environment where so much suffering and tragedy are regularly encountered. It serves a need to somehow diffuse the all-pervasive sense of futility that might otherwise occur. Gallows humor is actually healthy and provides not only some comic relief but also a bond between health care workers. However, there is a very fine line between this humor and humor that belittles or disrespects patients and their suffering. The latter is never acceptable and should not be attempted or tolerated. Appreciating a culture's unique humor is probably one of the biggest challenges for anyone entering a new culture, and the best course is often just to listen and not try to engage in attempts at humor until well settled into the new culture.

The Missions of American Medical Education

All institutions of medical education in the United States have a dual mission and, in some cases, a triple mission.

PATIENT CARE

The first mission is and must always be to provide effective, compassionate and safe patient care. This is achieved by adhering to the highest standards of evidence-based medicine and implementing proven protocols and treatment regimens. Medical education institutions are subject to tight regulatory control, and they are regularly scrutinized by organizations like the Joint Commission on the Accreditation of Healthcare Organizations (JCAHO).

MEDICAL EDUCATION

The second mission of medical education institutions is the education and training of physicians and other health care professionals who work, learn and train in them. Here too, there are very high standards for curriculum design, access to patient material, opportunity to participate in medical diagnostic and therapeutic procedures under appropriate supervision, faculty-to-trainee ratios, formal teaching, structured systems of assessment and feedback, and other components of a high-quality medical education environment. These are also subject to scrutiny by the Accreditation Council for Graduate Medical Education (ACGME), which periodically conducts in-depth on-site surveys of programs and interviews residents, faculty and key administrators. In addition to general institutional requirements, ACGME, through a system of specialty-specific Residency Review Committees (RRCs), establishes goals, objectives and requirements for training in each specialty. In addition to setting high standards, this ensures a level of consistency across programs within a given specialty throughout the country. Only programs meeting and maintaining standards set by ACGME can continue to function and recruit residents and fellows.

A third mission for some institutions that are privately owned and operated with the intention of yielding a profit is to have revenues exceed expenses. Although this is more consciously articulated in "for-profit" institutions, in reality no institution can long function if the reverse is the case (i.e., if expenses consistently exceed revenues). Revenues for a medical institution come primarily from medical insurers, the largest of which are the federal government via its Medicare program and state Medicaid programs, but revenues also include scores of private sector health insurance companies.

Roles of Residents

In popular American language, when someone is functioning in a certain role or discharging certain responsibilities, he or she is said to be "wearing a hat". When people must function in multiple roles or discharge multiple responsibilities simultaneously, they are said to be "wearing many hats". Consistent with the multiple missions of medical education institutions, residents also must wear many hats, and it is crucial that the newly arriving IMG be aware of his or her multiple roles.

PHYSICIAN

Just as patient care must be the first priority of the institution, effective, compassionate and safe patient care must also be the resident's first priority. Residents are first and foremost physicians who have responsibility for diagnosing and treating their patients by using the highest standards of evidence-based medicine applied conscientiously and with the highest professional standards. Without exception, the patient must always come first. However, residents, especially when first beginning their training, must be very aware of their limitations of both knowledge and experience and seek help from their senior residents, attending physicians or other appropriate health care professionals when they encounter situations beyond, or possibly beyond, their level of expertise.

STUDENT

At the same time, the resident wears the hat of a student. Only by assiduously applying himself or herself can the resident acquire the knowledge and skills necessary to actually provide quality patient care. Learning is a constantly ongoing process in residency and occurs not only in lecture halls and conference rooms but on rounds, in clinics and in operating rooms. The student physician needs to constantly learn throughout his or her residency and needs to learn how to learn. Self-directed lifelong learning will be required for the remainder of his or her career and good study habits, the ability to track down and access evidence-based information, and the ability to use patients as a stimulus for specific learning are essential skills to be honed in residency.

Another related hat that the resident wears is that of teacher. A core value in the tradition of medical professionalism has always been the willingness to take the time and effort to teach those less advanced, whatever the relative levels may be. Such a responsibility is in fact cited in the traditional Hippocratic Oath, which many American medical schools invite their graduates to take:

> "...to give a share of precepts and oral instruction and all the other learning to my sons and to the sons of him who has instructed me and to pupils who have signed the covenant and have taken an oath according to the medical law..."

Attendings teach senior residents, senior residents teach junior residents and junior residents are expected, even from the very beginning of their training, to teach medical students and other medical professional students. Often the most valuable learning comes from those only a single step ahead, those who best remember what it is like to not know or to know less. In addition, it is well recognized that one of the best ways to learn is to teach.

EMPLOYEE

Yet another hat the resident must wear is that of an employee of the institution. In that role he or she must be aware of the requirements to protect the institution from liability by adhering to established protocols and safety procedures, as well as the need to practice medicine as cost-effectively as possible. This may often be a challenge for the resident who may in some cases feel that more expensive tests or treatments are indicated than are available or being authorized by the institution or the medical insurers. The resident physician has a responsibility to advocate for the best possible care for his or her patient but at the same time must recognize the limitations of their ability to impact or change the health-care delivery system. Like so many other issues, the best source of guidance and information in such cases will generally be senior residents and attendings.

In addition to practicing cost-effective medicine, physician employees have a responsibility to adhere to institutional rules and regulations and comply with directives. Residents who are consistently remiss in tasks such as completing discharge summaries or submitting necessary forms and paperwork create work for others and may ultimately be subject to disciplinary actions. The institution pays the salary. It has the right to expect all employees, including physicians, to provide the services for which they are being paid and to exercise responsibility in helping the institution to be financially solvent and free of liability in order to continue providing care for its patients.

Summary

Many of the nuances of the multiple roles that the new IMG resident must play may be unfamiliar or different from those in their home medical institutions. The overall culture of American medicine, as well as the more subtle cultural aspects of training in various specialties or types of institutions, may also present challenges. Watchful observation, patience and a willingness to ask questions will ultimately be the best means of becoming comfortable in working and learning in the American medical system.

7 | Patient Care

Balu Athreya, MD, Hiren Shingala, MD, Vijay Rajput, MD,
Gerald P. Whelan, MD, Anuradha Lele Mookerjee, MD, MPH,
and Stephen S. Seeling, JD

Introduction — 97

Handling Relationships — 100

Relationships Between Patients and Physicians — 101

- Greeting and Conversation — 101
- Confidentiality — 102
- Examination Demeanor — 104
- Breaking Bad News — 104

Relationships Between Physicians and Family Members — 105

- Meetings with Patients and Families — 105

Relationships Between Trainees and Attending Physicians — 106

Relationships Between Trainees and Other Members of the
Health Care Team — 107

Relationships Between Physicians and Nursing Staff — 108

Other Allied Health Personnel — 108

- Case Manager — 109
- Clinical Nutritionist or Dietitician — 109
- Clinical Psychologist — 109
- Financial Counselor/Coordinator — 109
- Physical/Occupational Therapist — 109
- Radiation Technologist — 109
- Respiratory Therapist — 110
- Social Worker — 110
- Speech and Language Pathologist — 110
- Ward/Clinic Secretary — 110

Summary — 110

Daily Work Activities — 111

Patient Care Responsibilities — 111

- The Emergency Department — 112
- General Guidelines for Admitting New Patients — 112

▪ *Admission History and Physical*   114

▪ *Patient Management*   118

▪ *Presentation and Notes*   120

Being On-Call   126

▪ *Schedules*   126

▪ *The Night Float System*   127

▪ *Sign-Out Protocol*   127

▪ *Standard Duties and Responsibilities When On-Call*   127

▪ *Summary*   128

Working Outside the Residency Program   128

▪ *Moonlighting*   128

Medical Malpractice   130

What Constitutes Medical Malpractice?   131

Malpractice Insurance   132

Introduction

Balu Athreya

You are in a United States hospital, ready to start caring for patients. You have completed the requirements, improved your English-speaking skills, and gained a basic knowledge of the dual role of medical education, namely patient care and education of future physicians. You may not be familiar with all of the medical technologies available in this country, but you have experience caring for patients and working in a hospital in your country.

You are already aware that medical care is a combination of science, art, and high technology. In order to learn all about the science and technology of medicine, you have to take care of patients under supervision (Box 7-1) and with several other health care professionals (Table 7-1), which requires you to be able to work as one member of a professional team. This chapter deals with these human relations issues.

☑ **BOX 7-1   What is Supervised Training?**

■ Supervision is an important component of training in the United States, and the style may be different from several other countries. In this system, a junior physician learns to take care of patients from a more experienced clinician by a process of shared responsibilities. These responsibilities include making a diagnosis, devising a management plan, and carrying out the management decisions. The final authority is with the experienced clinician, the supervisor. Senior physicians take this responsibility seriously, and they are held accountable for their role as supervisors. The trainee is not free to make decisions and carry them out without consulting the supervisor, except in emergencies. However, he or she can make decisions as an exercise and anticipate what the senior supervising clinician is likely to do and thus learn.
■ In carrying out the management plans, the junior physician may have to perform technical procedures such as vascular access or lumbar puncture. Until he or she gets to be proficient, procedures are performed under the direct supervision of a senior trainee or the supervising physician. As the trainee proceeds to the second and third year of training and becomes competent in performing the procedures, he or she becomes the supervisor of the junior trainee. This gradual process of gaining experience under supervision and becoming independent is a particular strength of training in the United States. Supervised training plays a large role in surgical and radiology training. No trainee can perform surgery or a procedure on his or her own without the direct supervision of the attending surgeon or the radiologist.

Before getting into the specifics of the relationships in the hospital setting, some general remarks about the American personality and culture may be of help in understanding the dynamics of these relationships. These remarks are based on personal observation, reading of cultural anthropology, and feedback from several International Medical Graduates who completed their training in the United States.

It is important to remember that these observations represent modal or typical behavior of Americans as a group. There will be individuals who will not fit into this mold, particularly in the melting pot of America. It is also important to know that these modal behaviors change over time in every culture. Finally, these are not value judgments; these are documentations of how people think and behave. These attitudes to life's challenges are neither good nor bad, but there are strengths and weaknesses to these attitudes. (For more information, see the works by Kluckhohn and Spiegel in the Reference section.)

American culture still has a frontier spirit. The motto of the U.S. Army Corps of Engineers ("Seabees") says it best: "The difficult we do immediately. The impossible takes a little longer." The strength of this attitude is that it fosters an atmosphere in which man can go to the moon or manipulate the gene. There are some things, however, man cannot control, such as aging and death. In some respects, in America, even death is considered a failure. Therefore, these subjects affect the American psyche much more

TABLE 7-1	

List of Health Professionals

Title	Description*
Case manager	A health care professional who performs utilization review, coordinates admissions, and discharges and communicates with third-party (insurance) payers.
Clinical nutritionist	Master's degree with clinical fellowship experience.
Financial counselor	High school or college graduate with experience in accounting and able to work with patients and third-party payers.
Licensed practical nurse (LPN)	Assists nurses and nurse practitioners; also assists physicians. Certified after training in an accredited program, often a technical school.
Nurse practitioner	Master's degree and practical training; may work independently or under the license of a physician.
Occupational therapist	Graduate of an accredited program with a bachelor's degree or a certificate of proficiency.
Physical therapist	Graduate of an accredited program with a bachelor's degree or a certificate of proficiency.
Physician assistant	Graduate of an accredited school; assists physicians in medicine and surgery; cannot be independent.
Radiology technologist	An associate degree or graduate of an accredited training program; may have special training in one of the modalities such as ultrasound or CT.
Registered nurse	Graduate of an accredited school of nursing, with or without a bachelor's degree; may have trained in a specialty.
Respiratory therapist	Graduate of an accredited program; associate degree in respiratory sciences and clinical experience in respiratory care.
Social worker	Holds a master's or bachelor's degree; has clinical experience.
Specialty nurse	Registered nurse, specializing in one specialty under the supervision of a specialist physician.
Speech and language pathologist	Master's degree or a certificate of clinical competence and clinical fellowship experience.
Ward clerk/secretary	Performs a variety of tasks; ability to relate to people and computer skills.

*For detailed descriptions, go to http://www.ecfmg.org/acculturation and click on Interdisciplinary Health Care Team.

than in cultures that accept death and aging as part of nature. This almost adversarial attitude to death and aging helps to explain the inordinate efforts of many Americans to look younger and prolong life.

Americans are obsessed with time. The modal behavior of an American is to control it. Punctuality is emphasized; things get done on time, most of the time. Appointments are made months in advance. The negative side is that we cannot control time. Patient encounters are unpredictable, and it is impossible to keep to the allotted time in a regimented manner because some patients require more time. In addition, a physician's time is unpredictable because of emergencies that throw the appointment schedules out of control. However, patients take time off from work to come for appointments, and probably lose salary for taking time off. It is necessary to understand this factor and be prompt at the clinics. If you are going to be late, let the patient know ahead of time. At the least, apologize when you enter the room. The most common complaint about doctor's offices is the excessive waiting time.

An average American enjoys great individual freedom, and independence is encouraged from infancy. Many of the developmental problems of childhood and adolescence seen in this culture are related to pushing them before they are developmentally ready. This country is built on individual freedom and allows people to be the masters of their own fate, but it also comes with individual responsibility. Everyone is held responsible and accountable for the consequences of their actions.

In medicine, patients have their own Bill of Rights (see Appendix G). They also have responsibilities that go with the rights. For example, accident prevention is emphasized. Patients feel responsible for their own health. There is a movement to make patients, particularly those with chronic diseases, be more responsible for their own care. This puts great pressure on the individual. When things go wrong, this sense of responsibility leads to feelings of guilt, and when the guilt becomes unbearable, it is directed at the physician and the health care system.

One strength of this primacy of the individual is that decisions are made at the level of the individual or the small nuclear family. The negative side is that often there is no or little help from an extended family system, which leads to stress and the need for community support or services like counseling or social work.

In Chapter 5 of this work, you learned about "personal space", which is an essential component of the American personality. Personal space is related to the primacy of freedom and dignity of the individual, and it has legal implications, which is why "touching" issues were also emphasized in that chapter. Physicians have to touch "with care, concern, caution and compassion". It is polite and proper to inform patients before starting a physical examination, particularly with children. You do not want to touch any one without consent, even for a medical examination

Human dignity and dignity of labor are emphasized in this culture. The contributions of a sanitary worker, a secretary, and the division chief to the success of an organization are all equally respected, and each one of them also feels that what he/she does is important. The chief of a department will not consider it below his dignity to move a chair or throw out an overflowing trash bin. Once a physician is out of the work environment, he is one among many; there is no special pedestal for doctors, and the hierarchical system is less rigid. Physicians and members of the support staff, such as laboratory technicians or sanitary workers, interact much more easily in this culture than in many others.

Seniority and age do not have the same importance they are accorded in other cultures. Patients look for up-to-date knowledge, expertise, and trustworthiness in their doctors—not necessarily for gray hair. There is no need to call senior physicians as "sir," and they do not treat junior physicians like peons either.

The following relationships in a hospital setting will be discussed in this chapter in light of the characteristics of American culture as described in the earlier paragraphs:

- Patient and physician
- Physician and the members of the patient's family
- Trainee and the attending physician
- Trainee and other members of the physician team
- Physician and the nursing staff
- Trainee and members of the health care team

Fundamentally, all of these are *human* relationships.

Handling Relationships

Strong human relationship skills are essential to be successful in life—at home and at work. It is wonderful if you are naturally skilled in this area. It is certainly possible, and indeed essential, to develop these skills to be a good clinician, to be a good human being. Some of the skills that can be helpful are listed in Box 7-2. Remember that in the end, it is not how good you think you are in human relations, but the perception of the patient and others around you that matters.

☑ BOX 7-2   **Principles of Human Relations Skills: A Personal View**

- Genuine liking for people
- Genuine interest in helping others
- Being an excellent listener
- Remembering that everyone likes to be loved and recognized and no one likes to be pushed or ordered
- Able to see and respect another's point of view
- Being honest and truthful
- Not being afraid to say "I do not know" and "I am sorry"
- Being friendly and open
- Ability to express the facts truthfully and tactfully, without hurting, belittling, or crushing hope (knowing how to say what needs to be said)
- Ability to forgive
- A sense of humor
- Ability to accept others as they are and without judgment
- Avoiding arguments, at least in public
- Not forcing people into a corner, allowing room for others to save face

Human needs are the same all over the world. Patients' hopes, fears and expectations are the same in all cultures; however, there are four major modifying factors in the medical setting:

1. Being ill, particularly chronically ill, leads to suffering and to stress. Behavior under stress is unpredictable; therefore, patient behavior may not be understandable at times.
2. Cultural explanations of diseases and, therefore, expectations are different. Expressions of illness, called illness behavior, may not be what you were used to in your homeland.
3. There are some strict legal restraints on what you as a physician may and may not do. For example, you may not be able to give out information about a patient even to close relatives without the patient's written consent.
4. The payment system for medical care is based on a private practice model. Your attending physicians are paid specifically for every medical encounter. The patients may not pay directly, but a third party (i.e., an insurance company or the government) pays on their behalf. Therefore patients expect to have a professional relationship with the person whom they are paying for a service, which will affect the way you, as a trainee, interact with the attending physician and the patient. However, most patients are willing to let you learn through them under the supervision of their personal physician.

You may be working in one of several locations in the hospital such as inpatient units (including intensive care units) or outpatient clinics. You may work in an operating room (surgical trainees), an imaging unit (radiology trainees), or a research laboratory depending on the training program you have chosen. Some of your training may also be in a private practice setting. The principles of human and professional relationships will be the same, irrespective of the location, but the physical setting, available resources and expectations will be different.

RELATIONSHIPS BETWEEN PATIENTS AND PHYSICIANS

The physician-patient "dyad" is the pivot of medical practice. It is therefore essential for all physicians to behave in a professional manner and build a trusting relationship. Here are suggestions to develop a good relationship with patients.

Greeting and Conversation

1. Be professional, both in your actions and appearance. Simple but clean clothes with a physician's white coat will be correct for all occasions.
2. Introduce yourself as in this example: "I am Doctor Jones, and I am a junior resident. I work with Dr. Smith, and I have reviewed your records and medical information. I will be asking you some new questions and may need to clarify some information you have previously given to the emergency physician. I will also be doing some physical examination. After that I will be discussing my findings and thoughts with Dr Smith and we will let you know what we think is going on with you and give you our recommendations for further tests or treatment."
3. Address the patients by their last name (family name). Do not address patients with their first name. When addressing children, it is appropriate to use first names. Do not refer to patients as cases.
4. Verbal greeting with or without waving of the hand is appropriate for most occasions. It is not necessary to shake hands, unless the patient offers the hand first. This is particularly important with patients of the opposite sex. If you shake hands offer a firm but not uncomfortable, grasp of the hand; one or two up and down movements is sufficient, you should initiate letting go of the hand grasp. Hugging and touching of the cheeks are not acceptable.
5. Do not allow any room for accusation by patients of improper touching. You may not completely close the door when you are examining a patient of the opposite sex. When dealing with a female patient who does not have anyone accompanying her, make sure you have an observer, preferably a female nurse during physical examination. This is particularly important when examining the breasts and the genital area.
6. Speak slowly so the patient can understand your accent.
7. Similarly, ask the patient to speak slowly so you can understand the accents and idioms. If you have doubt, ask him to repeat the answer. At the end, summarize and ask for the patient's corrections.
8. Be punctual. Do not make patients wait. If you know you will be late, let them know. If not, apologize to them soon after introducing yourself. They will understand.
9. Patients feel that it is their right to receive a full explanation of all treatment options and to give input in the kind of care they receive. A Patient's Bill of Rights is given to patients by hospitals, and it will be wise for you to become familiar with it (see Appendix G). Patients are partners in decision-making, so make them better

informed so they can make informed decisions. Most patients are well informed because of the Internet and information technology. In addition, they want to know information specific and relevant to their condition. The majority of patients expect to be fully informed about all options and the corresponding pros and cons. This is a great time to educate patients. Explain the options, risks, and benefits in simple language. Do not use jargon or complicated statistics.

10. Although many patients are well informed, there are many patients who are not able to assimilate and follow basic medical instructions. Almost 50% of the population score low in health literacy, which is the ability to understand and effectively use basic medical information and instructions. Low health literacy can be seen in any ethnic group and at all educational levels; however, older patients, those from low socioeconomic conditions, recent immigrants, and those with chronic illness make up a large proportion of this group. At the least, each patient must be able to understand the physician's answers to three main questions: 1) What is my main problem? 2) What do I have to do? 3) Why is it important for me to do this? Some patients may not admit that they have trouble understanding the instructions because they feel embarrassed or ashamed or do not want to offend the doctor. Also, most of the written instructions given to patients are written at a higher level of literacy. Therefore, it is important that you help make your patient health-literate by creating an atmosphere in which the patient will not feel ashamed to ask "dumb questions". Use simple language, and employ visual media when appropriate. Ask patients to repeat what they have been told.

11. In order to be certain that patients can understand informational materials that they receive from their doctors, it is important that they be written clearly and simply. A fifth grade reading level is usually the target. Figure 7-1 shows a sample HEALTH TiPS information card prepared by the American College of Physicians Foundation. HEALTH TiPS are two-sided 4 by 6 inch sheets that are available in English or Spanish at http://foundation.acponline.org/hl/htips.htm.

12. Make sure to note any specific religious prohibitions or cultural taboos. For example, blood transfusion is not acceptable to followers of some faiths.

Confidentiality

1. Common sense and prudence dictate that personal health information should be kept confidential. Access to such information should be made available only to authorized individuals and even then, only the information necessary for the task at hand. Confidentiality is particularly important in this era of computers, the Internet, and the Health Insurance Portability and Accountability Act (HIPAA), which went into effect in 2001. You must become familiar with the requirements of this law, and you will be given training and an examination in the HIPAA before you gain access to medical records. This training is usually given during the orientation before starting residency. Familiarize yourself both with the HIPAA and the specific policies of implementation unique to your hospital.

2. Experienced, sensitive clinicians do not discuss patients in public places such as elevators or hallways. One has to be cautious about revealing the identity of patients, even during morning reports and classroom lectures, to abide by HIPAA regulations. It is generally acceptable to discuss details of a patient's illness with other members of the health care team, with consultants who are invited to advise on a patient, with a physician who will be assuming care immediately on discharge, or

FIGURE 7-1

Sample HEALTH TiPS information card prepared by the American College of Physicians Foundation. (HEALTH TiPS are available in English or Spanish at http://foundation.acponline.org/hl/htips.htm. Copyright © 2007 by the American College of Physicians Foundation.)

HEALTH TiPS
WHAT YOU CAN DO

Smoking

Smoking can make you sick and shorten your life. If you quit now, you will be healthier. Quitting is hard work, but there are ways to help you.

- Smoking is dangerous, especially if you already have heart or lung disease or if you are pregnant.
- It increases your chances of having a heart attack, stroke, lung disease and cancer. When you smoke, you can make people around you sick—even your children.
- You can quit smoking even if you have smoked for a long time.
- When you quit smoking, you will feel better, live longer and save money.

Ask Your Doctor

- Why it is important for you to quit
- How quitting can help you

Ask Your Doctor what help you can get to stop smoking.

- Ways you can help yourself
- Treatment groups with other smokers
- Medicines to help stop the urge to smoke

After starting your program, set up times to see your doctor. Next visit date:_____

AMERICAN COLLEGE OF PHYSICIANS
FOUNDATION

HEALTH TiPS
WHAT YOU CAN DO

Smoking

To help you fight the urge to smoke:

- Set a date in the next two weeks to stop smoking and stick to it.
- Throw away all your cigarettes and ashtrays.
- Stay away from other smokers.
- Tell your family and friends you are quitting and ask for their help.
- See your doctor to keep track of your progress.
- Talk to your doctor if you are having trouble, especially if quitting makes you gain weight or feel depressed.
- Stick with your plan.
- If you fail, don't give up. Try again. Some people need to start over three or four times before they beat the habit.
- For extra help, call 1-800 QUIT NOW.

For more information, go to **www.MedlinePlus.gov** and search for "Smoking."   © 2007 ACP Foundation

with immediate members of the family (unless the patient specifically does not want some members of the family to know about his or her condition). If persons from outside call claiming to be a member of the family or friend, you may let them know about the patient's general condition. If they want details, it is best to direct them directly to the patient or to a family member. If you have any doubts, check with one of your senior residents or supervisors.

☑ BOX 7-3 **Essential Elements of Communication in Medical Encounters**

1. *Build a relationship*: Build a strong, therapeutic, trusting relationship.
2. *Open the discussion*: Elicit the patient's full set of concerns.
3. *Gather information*: Listen actively; structure, clarify and summarize; use open-ended and closed-ended questions, as appropriate.
4. *Develop understanding*: Understand the patient's perspective.
5. *Share information*: Use language the patient can understand; check his or her understanding.
6. *Reach agreement*: Reach agreement on problems to be addressed and plans for treatment.
7. *Provide closure*: Ask for additional concerns; summarize and discuss follow-up plans.

From: The Kalamazoo Consensus Statement. Acad Med. 2001;76:390-3; with permission.

Examination Demeanor

1. The most important task is to develop a strong, trusting therapeutic relationship with the patient and the family. Effective communication and empathy are the key elements. Box 7-3 lists some of the essential elements of communication with patients.

2. Make sure you understand the patient's main concerns and priorities. At the end of the interview, summarize the major points you have understood.

3. Make sure the patient has adequate privacy during the examination. It is inappropriate to examine the patient in street clothes, particularly if you wish to get a good examination of the heart, skin, or musculo-skeletal system. Indeed you may miss important clues by doing so. It is appropriate to ask the patient to wear a gown or ask for complete exposure for some examinations. However, make sure there is someone else present during the examination, particularly if the patient is of the opposite sex.

4. At the end of the visit, once a plan has been formulated, describe the problem and solutions in simple language. Be truthful without either dashing hopes or falsely raising them. Do not be overly optimistic or pessimistic. What you say and how you say it matters, particularly because you are new to the culture.

5. If you do not know, say so. Tell patients how you plan to find an answer. Find the answer and get back to them on time.

Breaking Bad News

Breaking bad news is an essential skill to master. Honest disclosure about a patient's diagnosis allows the patient to make better informed health care decisions. The SPIKES approach is straightforward but also conveys empathy. It entails the following guidelines:

- *Setting up*: Breaking bad news should be done in private, by sitting down and making eye contact with the patient.
- *Patient perceptions*: Assessing patient perceptions allows physicians to correct misinformation and tailor the news to the patient's level of comprehension.
- *Invitation to break news*: Physicians need to get the patient's permission to share bad news.
- *Knowledge*: Physicians should convey information at the patient's level of comprehension.
- *Emotions*: Enough time should be given to the patients to vent their emotions.

■ *Strategy and summary*: Physicians can minimize the patient's anxiety by summarizing the areas discussed, checking for comprehension, and formulating a strategy and follow-up plan with the patient, after having given the bad news.

RELATIONSHIPS BETWEEN PHYSICIANS AND FAMILY MEMBERS

In most situations, someone accompanies a patient, and this is particularly true for patients coming in for admission, children, the elderly, and those with mental health problems. They may be a good source of history in some situations and a great source of support for the patient. However, privacy of patients is of paramount importance. Therefore it is necessary to know who the accompanying person is, what the relationship to the patient is, and whether the patient wants this person to be included in discussions. Do not assume that a member accompanying the patient is necessarily the spouse, parent, or offspring. Look at the chart before you enter the examining room so you can address them properly.

You should know the name of the person designated by the patient to be notified in case of emergency. This is usually the authorized legal contact or guardian. This is particularly important at the time of discharge of children, elderly, and those with mental illness.

In geriatrics, it is important to know who has the power of attorney. If a patient is too ill or too demented, you have to be sure who the authorized person is for making decisions. In some situations, you may have to get a court-appointed guardian to make decisions on behalf of the patient. When you encounter such situations, it is best to work with your seniors who know the hospital policies and procedures.

In pediatrics, biological parents are the legal guardians in most situations. In some situations, only one parent has legal custody and is authorized to give permission for treatment. The other parent may or may not be involved or sometimes not authorized to even visit. In some situations, there is no biological parent. An adoptive parent or a foster parent may accompany a child.

Irrespective of the family arrangements, your duty is to take good care of the patient and support his/her family through the stress. Good human relationship skills are applicable in all situations.

Meetings with Patients and Families

1. Use the guidelines summarized in Box 7-4 during conversations with patients and families.
2. After a conference with patients and families, document the actual events and transactions. Write the facts, not your opinions, interpretations, or judgment.
3. If you made an error, be honest and let the patient and family know. Also, make sure your supervisor/attending physician knows. Ultimately, he/she will be responsible for your error. Document the event according to the requirements of the institution and inform the risk management official. Every hospital will have someone in charge of risk management (Box 7-5).
4. You may sometimes encounter patients who are difficult to relate to. Do not start arguing with them, particularly in public places and corridors. Seek the help of senior colleagues or someone from the patient relations office (Box 7-6). Take the patient to a quiet place where you can have a calmer discussion. Have a third party, such as member of the social service department or nursing service, present.

☑ BOX 7-4   **Guidelines for Discussion with Patients and Families**

- Ensure privacy and adequate time.
- Assess what the patient already knows about the problem. Some information the patient provides will be correct but not all. This assessment will be a good lead into serious discussion.
- Provide honest information in simple language. Speak slowly so that the patient and the family members understand.
- Explain all the relevant facts. Patients expect to be informed fully, so share both good news and bad news. You must be truthful but not blunt. The way you convey the message and the words you choose matters. It is possible to give bad news without crushing all hope.
- Discuss all options. Give the advantages and disadvantages of the alternatives.
- Have a third-party present, if available and if appropriate. In some situations, it is necessary. This person may be a nurse, a social worker, or a clergyman.

Source: Girgis A, Sanson-Fisher RW. Breaking bad news: consensus guidelines for medical practitioners. J Clin Oncol. 1995;13:2449-56.

☑ BOX 7-5   **Risk Management**

- Many hospitals employ personnel called *risk managers* to initiate activities to prevent adverse patient outcomes.
- Risk management has evolved into a special field of hospital management, with focus on anticipating, analyzing, and controlling factors leading to adverse events in the entire system.

☑ BOX 7-6   **Patient Relations**

- Many hospitals have an office of community and patient relations. Its function is to provide patient advocacy and assist patients and hospital staff in resolving difficult and controversial issues.
- This office often maintains a list of language interpreters to help patients and doctors. It may also help coordinate community resources for patients.

Identify the problem and promise to bring it to the attention of your supervisor. Be sure to meet with your team and your supervisor, find a solution, and contact the patient for a follow-up meeting.

5. If a patient or a family member is disruptive, move him to a quiet place for a calm discussion. Do not aggravate the situation by arguing with the patient or getting physically too close. Make sure the person does not hurt himself or others. You may have to restrain the person or call a security guard. If so, you need to know the hospital policies and procedures. Often, the nursing supervisor or your senior can help you in such situations.

RELATIONSHIPS BETWEEN TRAINEES AND ATTENDING PHYSICIANS

Every patient admitted to the hospital or a clinic will have an attending physician. This may be a faculty member, a private physician, or a hospitalist physician (a physician who is responsible for inpatient care regardless of their specific appointment). The attending physician is the physician of record. This physician may be the same or different than the physician who cares for the patient outside of the institution, also known as the primary care physician or primary medical doctor. The attending physician is responsible for all diagnostic and management decisions, and he or she bears the ultimate legal responsibility for the outcome—good and bad. Everyone taking care of the patient, including the trainees, has moral, ethical, and legal responsibility, but the attending physician is the person who receives payment for care from the insurance company or other payers. He or she will have to justify the services provided and the charges for those services.

The attending physician is also responsible for teaching the trainees in medicine and allied health fields through his patients. In essence the trainees are allowed to learn by taking care of the patient at the pleasure of the patient and the attending physician. Patients are generally aware of this, particularly in teaching hospitals. Almost all of them know this is necessary for the training of future doctors and the welfare of the society. You may encounter few rare patients who do not want to be examined by trainees.

Make sure you introduce yourself as a trainee when you meet the patient for the first time. Inform the patient of the following: who the attending physician is and that you will be discussing all of the details with him or her; the attending physician will come in to talk and to examine; all decisions will be made in consultation with the attending physician. Attending physicians are required to examine each patient both in the hospital and in the outpatient departments, write their own brief notes, and countersign all of the orders written by the trainee.

Senior physicians do not bear down heavily on trainees and do not reject new and fresh ideas. Indeed they encourage younger physicians to show enthusiasm, develop new ideas and grow independent. You will find the attending physicians in the United States very friendly and approachable. They do not like to be addressed as sir or madam. Although it is common to hear trainees in senior years addressing the attending physicians by their first name, it is best to address your senior physicians respectfully with their title and last name (family name), such as "Dr. Smith," particularly in the presence of patients.

These teachers like trainees who think on their own and ask relevant and critical questions. They will let you develop a diagnostic strategy or treatment plan, listen to you, and use your plans as starting points for teaching. As you advance in your training and acquire a sufficient knowledge base and skills, they will let you make more and more decisions and perform procedures with supervision. This is particularly true if you also show enthusiasm, hard-working habits, human relations skills, and trustworthiness.

Also remember that the learning environment in the United States is heavily focused on compliance with administrative issues such as HIPAA, the 80-hour work rule, MEDICARE laws, and insurance regulations.

RELATIONSHIPS BETWEEN TRAINEES AND OTHER MEMBERS OF THE HEALTH CARE TEAM

In every training program, there will be trainees at several levels. All of these trainees will be under the supervision of a senior or a chief resident, who in turn will be working under the supervision of the attending physician. In addition, each team may include several medical students. Usually, the chief resident is the liaison with the attending physician.

In university medical centers and those with specialty training programs, there will be specialty residents (fellows) who may be the liaison between the patient care team and the attending or the consulting specialist. Be aware of the relationships and the line of communication because there are variations in the hierarchy. When in doubt, ask your senior.

The usual routine is for the trainee to work on a patient and present to the attending physician in consultation with the senior resident. The senior resident is expected to teach the junior resident and help with implementation of treatment plans, performance of technical procedures and management of emergencies. All treatment plans are approved by the attending physician except in emergencies (see chapter on work rounds).

When several consultants are involved in the care of a patient, it is important to keep communication lines open between the patient, the attending physician, and the floor team. A specialist consultant may recommend an investigation or treatment and write notes to that effect. Make sure you discuss with the attending physician before implementing, unless it is an emergency. It is the responsibility of the attending physician to receive the consults, prioritize them, and discuss them with the patient before implementing. You can help the process by reading the consults carefully, clarifying any doubts and conflicting ideas, and presenting them to the attending physician.

A new trend is to have hospitalist physicians, which has improved the efficiency and cost of care. Teaching also has benefited in some ways; however, the patient does not have as much continuity of care in and out of the hospital.

RELATIONSHIPS BETWEEN PHYSICIANS AND NURSING STAFF

In the United States, registered nurses (RNs) play a major role in health care delivery and are often great patient advocates; therefore, they are trusted and respected by patients and physicians. In addition to their traditional role in caring for patients and helping to implement care management decisions, they are deeply involved in patient education.

In this system, you as a trainee write the orders for management of the patient, based on discussion with your seniors and the primary physician. The nurses often carry out the orders, including inserting IV lines, Foley catheters, administering medications, etc. There may be variations between institutions and specific units.

Nurses who work in one specialty area are called *specialist nurses* (e.g., the neonatal nursery, the dialysis unit). They know the details of care and the hospital routines much better than your seniors in training and sometimes better than the attending physicians. Develop good relationships with them. You can learn a lot from them and they can be very helpful.

You may also work with licensed practical nurses (LPNs), graduates of technical school who work under the supervision of physicians and registered nurses. Their background and training are not as extensive as those of registered nurses.

You may work with nurse practitioners who are registered nurses who have gone through formal training and obtained a master's degree. They have to be licensed in each state, and they work under the medical license of specific medical practitioners. They can do many of the duties of a physician, such as performing routine history and physical examination, ordering laboratory tests, and routine prescription writing. If they work in a subspecialty, they may be able to perform duties such as starting insulin pumps, placing access for IVs, etc. The rules for their practice vary from state to state.

Physician assistants belong to a separate group. They are graduates of accredited programs and have to be licensed to practice. They can also see patients and assist in surgery, but they are not independent practitioners.

OTHER ALLIED HEALTH PERSONNEL

A list of other allied health personnel who will be part of your medical care team at some point during your training and a description of their roles are given below. Teamwork depends on communication and cooperation. Remember that conflicts and disagreements have to be discussed and resolved amicably, and that the patient is the priority, not your ego.

Case Manager

- Driven by the increasing cost of care, a new group of personnel, case managers, were added to many hospital staffs in the 1980s to bridge the gap between acute and chronic care and to minimize unnecessary admissions and prolonged hospital stay.
- This role expanded subsequently to include concurrent and retrospective utilization review ("a process for monitoring the use and delivery of services, especially one used by a managed care provider to control health care costs") of all inpatients, to communicate with third-party payers and physicians, to coordinate admission and discharges, to help with discharge planning, and to prevent under- and over-utilization of resources.
- Many case managers are nurses.

Clinical Nutritionist or Dietitian

- Plans food and nutrition programs; supervises the preparation of meals, particularly for patients with special needs (e.g., diabetes, renal failure); assesses patients' nutritional needs; and develops and implements appropriate diets.
- Is a graduate of an accredited program, often with a master's or bachelor's degree.
- Requirements for licensing and certification vary from state to state.

Clinical Psychologist

- Duties include interviewing patients, administering psychological tests, and providing individual, family, or group therapy and behavioral modification programs, but not prescribing medications.
- May consult with medical personnel regarding the best treatment.
- A doctoral degree (PhD) and licensing are required for independent practice. Some with a master's degree may work under the supervision of a psychiatrist.

Financial Counselor/Coordinator

- Main function is to bill for services properly and to provide liaison with insurance companies and third-party payers.
- In some institutions, may also help the patients and families with appropriate counseling.

Physical/Occupational Therapist

- Provides evaluation, treatment, and consultation to all patients under the prescription of a physician.
- Holds a bachelor's degree or a certificate of proficiency in physical or occupational therapy and has to be licensed.

Radiation Technologist

- Also known as a *specialist technologist* (e.g., ultrasound technologist, MRI technologist).
- Goes through a special technical training program to be certified and needs a state license to practice.

Respiratory Therapist

- Provides extensive services from evaluation of respiratory status to tracheostomy care and ventilator management.
- Graduate of special training programs in accredited institutions.
- Must have completed a national certifying examination and be licensed.

Social Worker

- Services provided differ in different institutions to help people function the best they can at home, including liaising with community services, counseling, helping patients resolve family relationships and personal problems.
- Requires a master's degree in social work from an accredited school and supervised experience. Some may specialize as in psychiatry or pediatrics.

Speech and Language Pathologist

- Holds a master's degree in speech and language pathology from an accredited university.
- Must pass an examination, serve a clinical fellowship year, and be licensed to practice.

Ward/Clinic Secretary

- A pivotal person on each floor and in outpatient clinics. Keep a good relationship with them. They will make your life easy.
- Performs a variety of tasks including receiving the patients to the floor/clinic, informing the doctors and nurses, maintaining the roster of patients, and managing supplies, etc.

Detailed information about the concept and function of the interdisciplinary health care team and the roles and responsibilities of its members can be found at http://www.ecfmg.org/acculturation.

SUMMARY

You must develop a good relationship with every member of your team and learn to communicate effectively with each and every one of them for the welfare of the patients assigned to your care. You will be spending a major part of your waking time with these professionals, and you may as well have a pleasant relationship with them both for your mental health and for the welfare of the patients.

Good human relationships involve several features, as outlined earlier. Respect for the individual, respect for the others' knowledge and capability, good listening habits, ability to communicate, reasonable control of emotions, a sense of humor, humility, and a sense and respect for your time and others' time are crucial in all human relationships, particularly at work.

Although there is a hierarchy in any medical team, everyone likes to be respected for what he or she does. Team members are proud of the work they do to help patients and you. Acknowledge their help and be a pleasant team member.

Remember that the new requirements for eligibility to take medical specialty certifying examinations include an evaluation of the ability of trainees to work with a team and professionalism. Evaluation forms will be filled out by some of the members of your team as part of your training requirements and will count when you apply to take the certifying examination.

Daily Work Activities

In U.S. teaching hospitals, patient care activities begin early each morning. PGY-1 residents (interns) are usually the first line of patient care. Nurses and any other members of the health care team will usually contact them first regarding patient care issues.

Upon arrival each morning, residents first should get "sign out" information from the night float team/cross covering team about any developments or problems with their patients. Work rounds are usually made first with residents and medical students, and teaching rounds with an attending physician take place later in the morning. After teaching rounds, residents usually attend an educational noon conference. In the afternoon, they may be involved with discharging patients, reviewing and implementing consults' recommendations, doing procedures or other patient care tasks. The whole team meets again later in the afternoon for sign out rounds. If not on-call, residents can then sign out to the on-call team and leave the hospital. A typical schedule of activities for a first-year internal medicine resident is detailed in Table 7-2.

TABLE 7-2

Typical Schedule of Activities for a First-Year Internal Medicine Resident

Time	Tasks
6:30 a.m. – 8:00 a.m.	Get sign out from night-float team/cross-covering team; note any acute issues; prioritize problems; see all patients.
8:00 a.m. – 9:00 a.m.	Work rounds with medical students and senior resident.
9:00 a.m. – 10:00 a.m.	Resident goes to morning report; intern finishes up work: calls consults, checks labs, finishes notes. In some programs, intern will also go to morning report.
10:00 a.m. – 11:45 a.m.	Teaching rounds with attending physician.
Noon – 1 p.m.	Core curriculum conference (noon conference). Lunch.
1:00 p.m. – 3:30 p.m.	Finish work/follow-ups; prepare papers for patients to be discharged next day; family meetings; call primary care physicians as appropriate.
3:30 p.m. – 4:00 p.m.	Sign out rounds with team. Some programs also use this time to have a resident or medical student briefly review a topic or journal article.
4:00 p.m. – 4:30 p.m.	Sign out to on-call team and leave.

Typical daily schedules vary depending on the resident's specialty and rotation as well as whether the resident is on-call that day, the number of patients assigned to the team, outpatient clinic schedules, special educational conferences and other factors. Surgical specialties usually round early in the morning with the whole team and spend most of their time in operating rooms during the day. Many programs have their core curriculum conference condensed into a half-day educational conference one day of the week.

PATIENT CARE RESPONSIBILITIES

Hiren Shingala, Gerald P. Whelan, and Vijay Rajput

Every residency must strike a balance between optimal patient care and education of housestaff. Patient care in the United States differs from that in many countries in that it is team based. It is essential that residents learn to work effectively with all members of the team (see the section on Handling Relationships above).

Responsibilities of interns/residents include, but are not limited to, the items listed in Box 7-7 and those described below.

☑ **BOX 7-7 Responsibilities of Interns/Residents**

1. Admission of new patients
2. Visitation and examination of all patients on your team each morning
3. Work rounds
4. Presentation and notes
5. Teaching medical students
6. Communication with other team members
7. Ordering appropriate labs and imaging studies
8. Ordering appropriate and early consultations
9. Follow-up and sign-out rounds
10. Discharge planning and discharge processing, including dictations
11. Medication reconciliation
12. Patient education

The Emergency Department

In the United States, most patients presenting to an emergency department (ED) are initially evaluated by physicians who are specially trained in emergency medicine. Their role is to stabilize the patient, initiate basic evaluation and treatment and arrange for admission to the appropriate service and level of care—for example, medicine, surgery, intensive care unit (ICU), coronary care unit (CCU), and general wards.

When ED physicians believe a patient warrants admission to any service, they contact the appropriate physician from that service or the resident on-call for the service. However, if patients have private physicians they will usually be contacted first. With respect to internal medicine, at some hospitals medicine attendings are the initial contact person, while at others it is the resident on-call. Some hospitals have a medical admitting resident (MAR) who is the contact person for all admissions to the department of medicine. Flow for admissions to services other than medicine (e.g., surgery, Ob-Gyn) follow similar patterns. Usually ED physicians need attending physicians to accept and admit patients to the hospital.

General Guidelines for Admitting New Patients

■ Review ED chart including resident and attending notes (history and physical examination), nursing notes, medications given, vital signs, oxygenation, pain assessment, laboratory evaluations, electrocardiogram (ECG), and imaging studies.

■ Obtain complete history directly from patient. Some patients may not be able to provide detailed or accurate information due to nature of illness, delirium, or dementia. In those cases obtain information from family members or a health care proxy if one is available. This is a very common scenario with critically ill patients (e.g., on mechanical ventilation), patients in a nursing home and geriatric patients.

■ Perform physical exam with detailed examination of pertinent organ systems.

■ Request and review old records, if available.

■ Determine level of care: general ward, telemetry, ICU, or CCU. If it differs from level of care determined by ED physicians, discuss with them and admitting attending and resolve before transferring the patient from the ED.

■ Always obtain name (and contact information if possible) of primary care physician because it will be crucial for future communications. The primary care physician, commonly referred to as family physician or family doctor in other parts on the world, provide the first contact for a patient with an undiagnosed health problem and continuing care of medical conditions. They are commonly trained in family medicine or internal medicine, but can be trained in pediatrics or Ob-Gyn.

■ Always get emergency contact information for a family spokesperson. This is extremely important in the event of in-hospital emergency situations.

■ Obtain a list of medications that the patient is taking at home and update the Medication Reconciliation Form. Get that information from the patient, family, primary care physician, pharmacy or last discharge summary. Pharmacies are a very helpful source of information for current medications and are often open 24 hours per day. If the patient cannot remember the pharmacy name or location, use the Internet to locate the pharmacy. This is a critical step to avoid duplication, improper dosing, and drug interactions. Details about the process of medication reconciliation are discussed later in this chapter.

■ Determine if the patient needs to be isolated for reasons of infection control. Table 7-3 summarizes the specific isolation recommendations for individual pathogens.

TABLE 7-3

Infection Control Precautions for Heath Care Institutions

Description	Indication
Universal precautions.	For all patients.
Airborne isolation—Patient isolated in a private room with negative air pressure; the door must remain closed, and all entering persons wear masks with a filtering capacity of 95%. Transported patients must wear surgical masks.	For patients with known or suspected illnesses transmitted by airborne droplet nuclei such as tuberculosis, measles, varicella, or disseminated varicella zoster virus infection.
Droplet isolation—Patient isolated in private room and hospital personnel wear face masks when within 3 feet of the patient.	For patients with known or suspected illnesses transmitted by large-particle droplets such as *Neisseria meningitidis* infections and influenza.
Contact isolation—Patient isolated in a private room or with patients who have the same active infection. Nonsterile gloves and gowns are required for direct contact with the patient or any infective material; gowns and/or gloves are removed prior to exiting isolation rooms.	For patients with known or suspected illnesses transmitted by direct contact including infections due to vancomycin-resistant Enterococci and methicillin-resistant *Staphylococcus aureus*.

■ Always ask every patient about their code status, power of attorney and advanced directives. If the patient has any of these documents, make sure there is a copy in the chart.
   a. Code Status: expresses patient's wishes in cases of cardio-respiratory arrest; typically expressed as full code (perform all medical interventions to restore cardiopulmonary function), DNR (Do Not Resuscitate), DNI (Do Not Intubate) or DNI/DNR.
   b. Power of Attorney: a surrogate medical decision maker for when the patient is not competent to make decisions, for any reason. The person with power of attorney makes decisions on behalf of the patient based on their understanding of what the patient would have chosen to do if they had been able to express

themselves. The decisions should not be based on the power of attorney's personal beliefs, but rather on the patient's wishes and beliefs.

c. Advanced Directives: an advanced directive is an official document prepared by the patient in advance of an incapacitating medical or surgical illness that specifies what kind of care the patient would like to receive if he/she is unable to make medical decisions. Usually references a specific medical condition or treatments such as mechanical ventilation, feeding tube placement, dialysis, blood transfusion, and end-of-life care.

■ If you cannot obtain information directly from the patient for any reason, obtain information from relatives, friends, or neighbors. Call patient's relatives if needed.

■ If patient has been transferred from an extended care facility (e.g., nursing home, rehabilitation center), they should have paperwork with them. Review that paperwork and contact the extended care facility if more information is needed.

■ Document all the information in admitting history and physical in the chart (see below), sign your note and write your beeper number. Some hospitals have electronic health records (EHR) and your documentation may need to be entered electronically (typed, using a keyboard).

■ If you are not going to follow the patient you are admitting, you must contact the receiving team and provide a sign out. This involves updating them about the patient in brief including the pertinent history and physical examination findings, important laboratory and imaging findings, your assessment and plan, current patient status, and issues to follow up.

Admission History and Physical

The admission history and physical (H&P) is one of the most important components of the inpatient medical record. Because it is also one of the first forms of documentation that the new IMG will be expected to complete, it deserves special attention. It serves multiple functions:

1. Providing a complete record of the patient's medical history including past and current medical problems, medications, and allergies
2. Documenting familial risk factors and social histories
3. Documenting patient's concerns or complaints and their relationships to known medical conditions
4. Documenting physical findings at the time of admission as well as results of laboratory studies, electrocardiogram, and radiological studies at the time of admission
5. Proposing a synthesis of subjective and objective data to identify problems, diagnoses, and differential diagnoses to develop diagnostic and therapeutic plans

Other than keeping subjective information in the history and objective information in the physical or "data" portions of the document, actually writing the H&P is a matter of individual style. Narrative writing in full sentences or entering data in "bullet" form are both acceptable, providing that the information is clear and complete. Each writer should develop their own style and be able to adjust their writing depending on the individual case.

The format of the H&P document varies from hospital to hospital and from one specialty to another. Some hospitals have no pre-specified format and specific content is at the discretion of the writer. Other hospitals have formatted paper H&P forms that outline the general categories with the specific data to be filled in for each category. An ever-increasing number of hospitals have fully formatted computer-based H&P documents as part of a comprehensive electronic health record.

Although a comprehensive H&P might seem to be desirable and ideal in all cases, experience has shown that some will not include all the desired elements. One practical reason is that the busy resident will not have the time to conduct a complete history and physical exam on a patient for whom many portions may not be relevant, nor the time to write such an exhaustive document. In addition, busy consultants may often skim over dense entries that contain too much information and find it difficult to identify the key important elements in the entry. So the admitting resident must exercise some discretion in selecting which areas to include and how much detail to provide while not neglecting sections and information that is critical for proper care and reimbursement; senior residents can clarify which these are and how to complete them properly.

There are many good standard texts that provide guidance, direction and examples of H&Ps, but most would give the following elements, in this order, as a basic outline. Where appropriate, issues that may be of particular concern to IMGs are also noted.

Source and *Reliability* of *Information*: whether from patient or family member, and how reliable the person giving the information appears to be.

- **IMG issue**—If there are significant language issues or the patient has a dialect that is difficult to understand, consider getting help from a hospital interpreter or at least noting the difficulty in the chart so others can be alerted that misinterpretations might have occurred.

Chief Complaint (CC): the main reason(s) the patient is being admitted to the hospital at this time, if possible stated in the patient's own words, which can then be marked with quotation marks.

- **IMG issue**—Patients may use terms or words that may be unfamiliar to the IMG resident. Be certain to clarify any term that is unclear. It is important to use the patient's own words rather than your interpretation of what the patient is saying.

History of *Present Illness* (HPI): a chronological account of how and when the present illness began and progressed, perhaps including reference to prior state of health.

- **IMG issue**—HPI should start off with patient's age and gender, and most would include race, particularly if it may affect the differential diagnosis (e.g., sickle cell anemia in a patient with anemia and pain).

Past Medical History (PMH): prior diagnoses, treatments, surgeries, hospital admissions that may have relevance to the present illness or the patient's overall state of health.

- **IMG issue**—It may be helpful to inquire specifically about diseases that are common in American patients (e.g., high blood pressure, diabetes, heart disease). These questions should be posed in lay terms when possible (e.g., high blood pressure rather than hypertension).

Medications (Meds): all medications that the patient is taking and dose and frequency.

- ■ **IMG issue**—Many Americans take over-the-counter (OTC) medications and/or herbal remedies that they do not consider as drugs and may not report unless specifically asked, "Do you take any medicines that you buy without a doctor's prescription or any herbs or supplements?"

Allergies (All): any medications, foods or substances that have produced allergic reactions; include a brief description of the reaction.

- ■ **IMG issue**—Many Americans use the term *allergic* for any adverse effect from a drug or food. They may say they are allergic to codeine when they really only experience gastric irritation or some other side effect; the acceptable abbreviation for no allergies is NKDA (no known drug allergies).

Family History (FH): age, health, and medical conditions of parents and siblings, as well as any common diseases that run in the family or are clearly inheritable.

- ■ **IMG issue**—Family structures in the United States are varied and include many single parents and many same-sex couples raising children. Do not assume relationships! Information about the health of extended family members may be more limited than what you expect.

Social History (SH): elements of patient's circumstances that may have a bearing on current illness or on treatment or disposition options. Consider including occupation, marital status, support systems and other relevant factors.

- ■ **IMG issue**—Many physicians include use of alcohol, tobacco, and "recreational" drugs here but they may better be addressed as a subheading of "Habits." Getting reliable information in this area can be challenging, and it may be important to stress the confidentiality of the interview and to ask in a nonjudgmental way. Many patients may falsely deny or under-report use of alcohol or drugs.

Sexual History: whether patient is sexually active with opposite or same sex partners, how many partners, and whether "safe sex" is practiced (e.g., use of condoms, birth control).

- ■ **IMG issue**—This can be a difficult area to broach with patients, and not only for IMGs. Some discretion can be exercised with patients who are obviously not sexually active or in whom sexual activity has no relevance to current illness (e.g., an elderly patient with a stroke). However, do not be surprised to learn such impressions can be wrong, so when in doubt, ask.

It is helpful to preface questions about sexual activity by advising the patient that such questions are routine and posed to all patients. And while it is important to address issues of unsafe sex, it is important not to express judgments regarding a patient's sexual preferences. Here again, stressing confidentiality is critical. An acceptable, nonjudgmental way of asking this question is, "Do you have sex with men, women, or both?"

In the case of transgendered patients be careful to determine how they prefer to be addressed (i.e., Mr. or Miss).

Review of Systems (ROS): report of physiological systems (cardiovascular, respiratory, etc.) that may be relevant to the current illness or to any ongoing health or medical problems the patient may have.

- **IMG issue**—This is probably one of the most variable parts of the history with respect to length and detail; where relevant, it is important to record pertinent negatives (e.g., "denies exertional chest pain"), particularly if this is helpful in "ruling out" conditions in the differential diagnosis.

Physical Examination (PE): portions of the physical examination that are relevant to the patient's current illness or to any ongoing medical problems.

- **IMG issue**—The vital signs may be found on nursing notes or elsewhere but should also be included in the H&P, especially if any are abnormal. Although they may not be strictly indicated in a given patient, it is best to include at least a brief heart and lung examination in all patients. When doing pelvic, GU, rectal, or female breast examinations, a chaperone (nursing attendant) should be present and the patient's modesty and comfort must be considered and respected. Nursing staff can provide the best guidance regarding chaperones and should be consulted. When these parts of the exam are not indicated they may be listed as "deferred" but if relevant should be completed later on.

Data: a listing of the results of any available laboratory work, imaging studies, cardiograms, or other diagnostics.

- **IMG issue**—This information may come from the emergency department or from the patient's primary care physician. Querying the hospital information system for lab data or radiology studies should reveal any studies already done. Comparison with prior data is important, and official and preliminary interpretations need to be documented clearly.

Assessment: a listing of the patient's known and possible diagnoses and problems.
Plan: diagnostic studies to be obtained and treatments to be initiated.

- **IMG issue**—There are many ways of composing these final but critical sections. Some list all assessments, then all plans. Others provide the relevant part of the plan with each assessment. However these are addressed, the critical point is that a consultant or other reader should have a clear idea of the admitting resident's impressions and management plans at the time of admission.

All assessments should reflect cognitive thought processes and be documented in the plan of care. Avoid words like "rule out" in the listing of the differential diagnoses. Prioritize life-threatening conditions first in the plan of care. Documentation of discussion with attending or senior level resident is important for good communication and for medicolegal purposes as well.

Patient Management

For All Patients

■ Generate an active problem list for the chart and one that can be carried with you.
■ Get sign-out data (events that transpired during the night, new data, patient status) from the night float or the last team covering your patients.
■ Prioritize the order in which patients need to be seen. Acutely ill patients are seen first, followed by new patients, complex patients, patients ready for discharge, and then chronic stable patients.
■ Develop a systematic approach to evaluating and collecting information about patients on your prioritized list (Table 7-4).

TABLE 7-4	

Systematic Approach to Data Collection

Data Collection Sources	Examples
Care giver	■ Patient's nurse
Charted information	■ Nursing notes ■ Last progress note ■ Consultations and consultation notes ■ Notes from allied health professionals (physical therapy, speech therapy, respiratory therapy) ■ Order sheet
Laboratory and other studies	■ Laboratory data ■ Imaging data ■ Electrocardiograms, rhythms strips
Patient	■ History since last seen and focused physical examination

---

■ Generate a problem-based 'To Do' List for that patient; for example, if an X-ray needs to be followed up for Mr. Jones, you can write that next to Mr. Jones' name on the patient list you are carrying. Do this for every patient on your list, and you will have a 'To Do' list at the end.
■ Contact the senior resident on service with any urgent issues regarding patient management for help and advice; otherwise, wait until work rounds.
■ Start acting on the 'To Do' list after work rounds.
■ All patients seen by medical students must also be seen by either an intern or senior resident. Housestaff must write their own progress notes on patients seen by medical students. Medical student's notes on hospitalized patients are not legal documentation of patient care but their notes need to be critically appraised by you for educational purposes.

For Patients New to the Team (New Patients Whom You Did Not Admit and Transfers from Other Units/Team)

■ Review ED events if applicable.
■ Confirm findings of history and physical and be prepared to present patient case on rounds.

- Clarify pre-admission medication list and update Medication Reconciliation Form accordingly.
- Clarify code status, advanced directives, power of attorney.
- Get old records to floor.
- For all patients arriving as transfers from other hospitals, review hospital course from referring facility in detail and summarize as part of the history and physical examination document.
- For ICU/CCU transfers review the transfer note and develop a problem list and a "to do" list. Always evaluate need for central venous access lines and Foley catheters and discontinue it if no longer indicated. Infections from such devices are a major source of increased morbidity and mortality.

Work Rounds

Most training hospitals employ work rounds led by the senior resident on the team. The goals of resident work rounds are both educational and patient care, including:

- Increasing resident autonomy to make decisions about the patient care plan.
- Developing and enhancing leadership, managerial and teaching skills.
- Allowing daily work to begin earlier (evaluation and management orders, consultations). This helps to deliver patient care more efficiently and permits timely discharge of patients.
- Allowing for more efficient teaching rounds with attending physician.
- Meeting ACGME expectations for separating work rounds and teaching rounds.

During the work rounds, the resident and student team "see" each patient at the bedside. Interns or students present a brief overview of what has transpired in the last 24 hours, summary of consultation reports, most recent laboratory and imaging results, an assessment, and a plan for the day. The resident modifies the plan, if necessary, and the team then moves on to the next patient. Acutely ill patients are seen first. If an interesting physical finding is noted, it is reviewed with the students and interns. Team leaders may use various teaching methods to emphasize practical clinical points.

Guidelines for Senior Residents for Work Rounds

- Rounds should start and end on time.
- Goals for each day's rounds are expressly stated and modified as appropriate for the day.
- For efficiency's sake, avoid checking labs, writing orders, or calling consultants during work rounds; this type of work is best left for after work rounds, but before teaching rounds if possible.
- Patients are seen during work rounds. This is the time for the senior resident to see each patient, listen to their concerns, and make a personal evaluation of each patient's clinical condition.
- Interns and students introduce their patients to the team with a brief description of the patient's clinical condition and reason for admission (e.g., "Mr. Jones is a 54-year-old male with diabetes mellitus and hypertension admitted with community-acquired pneumonia.").
- Consider presenting the patient's case at the bedside with the patient in attendance. This is an efficient use of time and allows patients to contribute missing

information and ask questions. Discretion should be exercised in discussing sensitive issues or things that may upset the patient.

- Every member of the team should always use disinfecting hand gel before and after each patient, whether or not anything was touched in the room.
- Always observe infection control procedures, which may include donning gowns, mask and gloves and use of a dedicated stethoscope and blood pressure cuff.
- Focus work rounds on the basic evaluation and management issues of patient care (e.g., Does the patient need a Foley or central venous access line? Are intravenous fluid orders appropriate? How is the patient tolerating therapy?).
- Address patient concerns. Explain the plan for that day (including anything that may happen to the patient) and address patient questions.
- Care for the learners. Demonstrate physical exam findings and give brief feedback on the spot.
- Make a plan for each patient and make sure all members of the team are comfortable with what will be presented at attending rounds.
- Team-building should be emphasized by including all members in the discussion of each patient.
- Ensure that students have practiced their presentations before presenting to an attending.
- Wrap up at the end of rounds and make a concrete plan for how and when attending rounds will be conducted.

Work rounds can significantly cut down the time needed for teaching rounds with attendings and allow for a more focused, problem-based discussion. If the attending prefers an alternate patient care plan, the team can then discuss it. This system gives the resident the autonomy and authority to become a true team leader while ensuring review by the attending who has ultimate responsibility.

Presentation and Notes

Presentation

Typically, three or four teaching cases are selected by the senior resident on the team to be presented by students or interns during teaching rounds. Here are some general guidelines for presenting a case during teaching rounds:

All daily presentations should be in the SOAP (Subjective, Objective, Assessment, Plan) format:

- *Subjective*: This is the initial part of the presentation, which includes subjective symptoms as described by the patient; it is the patient's history.
- *Objective*: This includes objective findings including results of the focused physical exam and laboratory data and other studies obtained in the past 24 hours.
- *Assessment*: This part includes a prioritized problem list, and, when appropriate, a differential diagnosis for undifferentiated problems.
- *Plan*: This includes a management plan for each problem. It may include, but not be limited to, new medications, changes in medications, additional lab or radiology tests, and required consultations. The last part of each plan is the disposition. Anticipated discharge date, mobility, home care needs or placement needs, and transportation to home and to follow-up appointments are factors to be considered in determining a disposition.

- Include pertinent positive (to rule in) and negative findings (to rule out) in your presentation.

The presentations are more detailed for new patients and become more concise and focused as active issues are resolved. Usually, it is the task of the senior resident on the team to update the attending about patients who are not presented formally in teaching rounds. This occurs at the end of teaching rounds.

Notes

Daily progress notes are one of the important tasks in a resident's day. The main purpose of the notes is documentation of findings, patient assessment, medications/treatments, and other communications to others caring for the patient. General guidelines for the daily notes are given below:

- Every patient must have a progress note each day, completed before the end of the day.
- Every progress note must have the patient identification on it (i.e., label/sticker).
- Every progress note must be signed, dated and timed. Your printed name and beeper number must be noted at the end.
- We suggest that your progress notes follow the SOAP concept (see above). Most progress notes include the following items: vital signs for the last 24 hours, results of laboratory and imaging studies, and updated medication list. Daily progress notes are not only important for effective communication but for utilization management and reimbursement by insurance companies. They are a legal record of patient care.
- It may be best to document the assessment and plan after morning teaching rounds to ensure they are valid and up to date.
- Address disposition status in all notes.
- Any new events or communication with the patient needs to be documented. *If you do not document what you did, it is as if it were never done.*

Teaching Medical Students

Most teaching hospitals have medical students as a part of the team. Teaching medical students is an integral part of residency training. Here are some guidelines for teaching students:

- Accompany medical students in their patient encounters to observe their interview and physical exam techniques.
- Allow enough time for assisting students with organizing clinical thoughts (creating a prioritized problem list), arriving at an assessment and plan, reviewing the student's progress notes, and practicing presentation skills.
- Feedback is an important part of day-to-day teaching (see Chapter 9).

Communication with Other Team Members

Communication amongst the team members is extremely important. This includes communication between medical students, residents, the attending, nurses, subspecialist consultants, the physical therapist, the social worker, the home care coordinator, and the case manager. The senior resident on the team plays a key role in fostering communication between different team members. Here are few things for the senior resident to note:

- Identify the learning goals/objectives, responsibilities, and expectations of each team member at the beginning of rotation.
- Explicitly identify the responsibilities of the members of your team, and update/reinforce them on a daily basis as necessary.
- Obtain pager numbers and other contact information of team members.
- Obtain the schedules of all members of your team and identify any conflicts and factor this into the daily management of your team.
- Be aware of all residents' outpatient clinic responsibilities. If there is a conflict (i.e., if two or more residents have clinic on the same day), it should be identified and resolved before the beginning of the rotation.
- Communicate with the team and attending physician on a daily basis.
- Determine who will call families, consultants, and the primary care physician.
- Provide an update of all patients' clinical status.
- Communicate with nurses and the case manager about the plan of care on a daily basis.
- Communicate with consultants about recommendations. Speak to the consultant directly about their recommendations. This can provide an excellent learning experience.

Appropriate Labs and Imaging Studies

- Inform patient about laboratory and other studies that you are ordering and why they are being done, including risks and benefits.
- Order only those tests clinically indicated: avoid standing lab orders unless warranted; think how or if the test will change management.
- Review pending imaging/study orders from transfers: discontinue those no longer warranted.
- Review all higher level (e.g., invasive, expensive, complex) studies with team/ resident before ordering: this includes studies requested by consultants.
- Consider allergies to radiocontrast dyes and renal function when ordering imaging studies.

Appropriate and Early Consultations

Given the increasing complexity of patients, it is not uncommon to have 1-2 (sometimes even more) consultants who are following or co-managing your patient. Here are a few things to note about consultations:

- Every consultation should be called personally. Always request the consultant to call back to discuss the results.
- When ordering consultations, formulate specific questions with the assistance of the team before calling.
- Try to call the consultants for new consults early in the morning (after work rounds). This helps them to organize their day and prioritize the consults.
- Ideally, consultants should be asked not to write orders on patients before discussing the orders with the primary team. This avoids duplicate testing and sometimes even adverse events.

■ Every consultation is a teaching opportunity for consultant and learning opportunity for residents.

Follow-Up and Sign-Out Rounds

Usually after the noon conference, interns/residents follow up on issues that were raised during work rounds or teaching rounds. They

- ■ Review results of laboratory and other studies
- ■ Review old records
- ■ Participate in family meetings
- ■ Perform procedures
- ■ Prepare discharge papers for next day
- ■ Follow up on consultation reports

Daily activities on floors end with sign-out rounds. Due to duty hour regulations for residents, the number of transitions in patient care has increased. So, when you are gone from the hospital, a different team of residents, the covering team, will be cross-covering your patients for any acute issues. For optimal patient care, you need to sign out your patients to the covering team. This includes a brief description of each patient with important events in their hospital course, events from today, any anticipated problems with suggestions for managing them, and issues to follow up. Some hospitals have electronic sign-out, but it is extremely important to sign out verbally as well.

Discharge Planning and Discharge Process Including Dictations

- ■ Discharge planning begins on the day of admission, not on the day of discharge. The date of anticipated discharge should be identified on admission based on previous experience with the same illness or disease. Interns can get help from the senior resident and attending on this matter.
- ■ Clarify insurance coverage. Case managers and social workers can help with patients who do not have insurance coverage.
- ■ Clarify patient's prescription drug plan. If the patient does not have one, get help from the social worker. Some pharmacies, such as Target and Wal-Mart, have discounted prescription plans for which a patient might qualify.
- ■ If you are planning to discharge a patient who is on opioids, call the patient's pharmacy and verify the last opioid prescription.
- ■ Assess mobility and acute rehabilitation needs, especially in the elderly population. Determine whether a formal evaluation by a physical therapist and/or occupational therapist is indicated.
- ■ Assess the need for home care. Patients who may need home care and visiting nurse services include
  1. Patients going home on intravenous antibiotics
  2. Patients who need frequent dressing changes
  3. Patients going home with drains
  4. Patients newly started on insulin
- ■ Evaluate acute or subacute rehabilitation and placement needs early. If you anticipate a need for placement into a rehabilitation center or nursing home, involve case managers and social workers earlier in the hospital stay rather than on the

day of discharge. This helps to expedite the process and decreases delayed discharges.

- Schedule follow-up appointments with the primary care physician and subspecialist consultants.
- Arrange for follow-up laboratory tests (e.g., INR in patients going home on warfarin). Make sure the results are sent to the primary care physician.
- Fill out discharge instructions 1-2 days before the anticipated discharge date. Do not wait until the day of discharge because that could lead to a delay in discharge and a dissatisfied patient and family members.

Discharge Summaries

Discharge summaries are one of the most important components of the discharge process. It is an important mode of communication with the primary care physician, to whom it provides discharge diagnoses, discharge medications, a brief description of the hospital course and pertinent data.

Discharge summaries are usually dictated. Residency training programs have varying policies about whether interns or senior residents complete the discharge summary and about the deadlines for their completion. Ideally they should be dictated on the day of discharge when you still remember the patient.

Components of a discharge summary are outlined below:

1. Name of dictating physician: state and spell name
2. Patient's name: spell
3. Patient's date of birth
4. Patient's medical record number
5. Admission and discharge dates
6. Primary care physician: state and spell name
7. Principle diagnosis at discharge
8. Other important diagnoses
9. Discharge medications: state name of medicine, dose and duration (if applicable)
10. Discharge instructions: follow-up appointments, pending lab tests and other studies, outstanding issues at discharge, diet and activity.
11. List discharge condition such as
- Ambulatory
- Non-ambulatory
- Asymptomatic
- Baseline
- Symptoms minimized
12. HPI
13. PMH
14. Medications on admission
15. Drug allergies
16. Pertinent social history
17. Pertinent physical exam on admission
18. Hospital course by major discharge diagnoses (problem-based) including:
    - All major laboratory, imaging procedure, or pathology results
    - Consults

▪ Procedures in hospital
▪ Complications in hospital

At the end of the discharge summary, identify who should receive copies of it (e.g., primary care physician, consultants). Spell names correctly and give addresses if possible. Typically, discharge summaries should be 1 to 1.5 pages but should never exceed more than 2 pages.

If a patient expires in the hospital, the discharge summary is replaced by a dictated expiration note. It is a brief explanation of the patient's presentation, hospital course and events leading to expiration.

Medication Reconciliation

Medication reconciliation is the process of comparing a patient's medication in the hospital to all of the medications that the patient has been taking at home. It is a crucial process to avoid medication errors such as omissions, duplications, dosing errors, or drug interactions. It should be done at every transition of care in which new medications are ordered or existing orders are changed (e.g., on admission, on discharge to home, on transfer to another facility).

Most of the hospitals have a Medication Reconciliation Form for this process. It could be electronic or on paper. Here are the steps for this process:

1. Develop a list of current medications
2. Develop a list of medications to be prescribed
3. Compare the medications on the two lists
4. Make clinical decisions based on the comparison
5. Communicate the new list to appropriate caregivers and to the patient.

Failure to reconcile medications may be compounded by the practice of writing orders, such as "resume pre-op medications," which are highly error prone and are known to result in adverse drug events. "Resume previous meds" should never be written on discharge papers.

Patient Education

Patient education is an important element of quality health care. The goal is to keep patients informed and involved in their care. All information, whether verbal or written, must be given at the most basic reading level. For patients who do not speak English, provide information in their native language, if possible. Place copies of educational material in their charts.

Patients should be educated daily about their problems, test results, diagnosis and updated plans for their care. The bulk of the patient education occurs at the time of discharge. There are multiple components involved in educating the patient at discharge:

▪ *Disease-specific education*: Most hospitals have written instruction booklets that should be given to patients depending on their diagnoses. At the same time, disease-specific facts should be emphasized verbally as well.
▪ *Medication use/changes/indications*: Patients must be educated about new medications, why they need them, how to take them, and any changes in their medications. Some medications may require demonstration (e.g., use of an inhaler). At

the same time, patients should be educated about the importance of adherence to medications. Also address potential side effects and what to do if they occur.

- Patient education should also include counseling regarding diet, exercise, and life style.
- Finally, be sure that the patient is aware of all follow-up appointments and any lab tests or imaging that has to be done after discharge.

Although physicians have primary responsibility for patient education, it is best done by involving all appropriate team members: attendings, nurses, dietitians, physical therapists, etc. The bulk of discharge education is usually done by nursing and ancillary staff.

Each patient's final diagnoses and prognosis should be confirmed with the attending and the team before discussion with patients.

BEING ON-CALL

Anuradha Lele Mookerjee and Vijay Rajput

To be "on-call" means to be immediately available to respond to patient care issues. Residents may be on-call within the hospital or may take calls from home or elsewhere provided that they can be immediately contacted by cell phone or beeper and can respond in an appropriate time period. The nature of call varies by specialty and level of training and may be every third or fourth night depending on the program. All residency programs must comply with work hour limitations that restrict the duration and frequency of call within an 80-hour work week.

The intern is usually the first to be called by the nursing staff when a medical question needs to be addressed. The next in the hierarchy is the second-year or senior level resident whom the intern consults for advice. The senior may either work side by side with the intern (particularly true early in the academic year), or allow the intern more independence. At all times, the senior resident must maintain close supervision of the intern while simultaneously helping the intern to become more independent in the decision-making process.

The resident on-call has a great deal of responsibility but should keep in mind that there are senior residents as well as fellows who are also on-call, some in the hospital and some through their beeper, who can be easily reached for any advice. Finally, the attending on-call can be reached by phone for any problems encountered during the on-call hours by the house staff. The attending may be a hospitalist who is in hospital, or one who is on-call by beeper and hence can be reached by phone.

Most hospitalists are pediatricians or general internists. These are attending level physicians whose practice is confined to supervising all facets of inpatient care delivered in the hospital by the housestaff.

Schedules

Every residency program has specific rules on the number of patients that each resident can manage on their service. For example, in the medicine residency training program, each resident is restricted to a maximum of twelve patients. The Accreditation Council for Graduate Medical Education (ACGME) has mandated nationwide restrictions on resident work hours. The current requirement mandates an 80-hour weekly limit, averaged over 4 weeks, with at least 10 hours of rest between duty periods. It places a 24-hour limit on continuous duty and requires that 1 day in 7 be free from all patient care. It also limits in-house call to no more often than once every third night.

When on-call, it is important to find time to rest even if it is only for a few minutes. The house staff is provided with on-call rooms which have the basic amenities necessary for on-call duties. The general cafeteria of the hospital provides meals for the housestaff on-call. A rested and fed resident functions more efficiently, and it is crucial to make time to meet these needs.

The Night Float System

There are various types of call systems for the different departments. In the night float system, all residents who work during the day leave in the evening and are replaced by a team that works from early evening until the following morning. There are various models with different time frames for starting and leaving the hospital. Typically the night float intern comes in at 8 pm to relieve the person who has been on-call during the evening, and stays till 8 am when the day team signs in. Usually the residents assigned to the night float system work in 2-week block rotations. Many training programs have now instituted the night float system.

The disadvantage of the night float system is that there is a risk of missing important information during the handoff from one team to another. Also, because this is night shift work, it may lead to work-related sleep disorders. One of the newer developments developed by emergency medicine and the pediatrics programs is a day float system. This team typically comes in at 12 noon and stays till the early night, thus offloading some of the day work, including the evaluation of new hospital admissions.

Sign-Out Protocol

With the different call systems in place, it is imperative that the resident learn to sign out in an effective manner. *Sign-out* is the hospital term related to transfer of information between teams caring for the same patient. The quality of transfer of care and the frequency with which it occurs can affect patient care. Different strategies can be employed to ensure adequate communication of critical information. One of the protocols developed by the Institute of Healthcare Initiatives involves the ISBAR methodology. This entails the following steps:

- I—Introduction: introduce oneself and then the patient
- S—Situation: state the patient's current condition
- B—Background: relate any relevant social or family issues
- A—Assessment: give your assessment and differential for the condition
- R—Recommendations: provide your recommendations for care

Standard Duties and Responsibilities When On-Call

Whatever call system is in place in your program, the basic protocol remains the same. As a physician in training, it is essential to maintain professional behavior at all times. It is also important to develop good communication skills with all members of the team. Learning people's names and greeting them on every occasion can go a long way. When in doubt regarding any issue, always turn to the senior resident or the attending for direction. If a patient or any of the other staff members treats you in an inappropriate manner, always turn to your attending for guidance.

When on-call you may often get overwhelmed with a lot of phone calls. It is imperative to prioritize and handle any acute crisis immediately by going to the patient's bedside. Many of the other routine requests can be handled over the phone. One should bear in mind that a simple chart review can help immensely in bringing about superior patient care. An important pearl to remember is that the intern is never alone. The senior resident, the nurse managers and the floor nurses all have a great role to play in smooth functioning of the system. Hence, it is prudent to turn to them for advice and direction.

Transferring a patient to critical care services like ICU or CCU calls for early identification of unstable patients who will benefit from early aggressive intervention and prevention of adverse events. When in doubt, always call the senior. Timely documentation of events is highly important. Records should reflect all services provided in real time. This includes receipt of critical lab values, responses to nurse's requests, family meetings, responses to patient's wishes and the like. This habit should be ingrained from the very beginning of internship training and is crucial for the efficient flow of patient care.

Summary

In the final analysis, being on-call is a great learning experience. It is the one special occasion when all the different facets of your training are put to use. It is also a special time of professional development that you will always remember.

WORKING OUTSIDE THE RESIDENCY PROGRAM

Anuradha Lele Mookerjee and Vijay Rajput

Moonlighting

Moonlighting is defined as any professional activity arranged by an individual resident that is outside the course and scope of the approved residency or fellowship program, whether or not the resident receives additional compensation. Moonlighting is prevalent among all residents and fellows in training in United States. The American Medical Association estimates that up to 37% of all residents moonlight, and the American Osteopathic Association believes up to 80% of residents in osteopathic programs moonlight. For internal medicine residents, educators say, the number is probably closer to 50%.

Moonlighting that occurs within the residency program and the sponsoring institution is termed internal moonlighting and is counted toward the 80-hour weekly limit on duty hours. As a trainee, your performance in the residency program must have your highest professional priority at all times. You must be available, alert, and fully responsible for all of the program's clinical and training activities; no activities outside the scope of the training program should interfere with these learning opportunities and their attendant service responsibilities. Given the clear priority of training, the leadership of each program decides whether its training requirements are compatible with moonlighting. The program director has the right to prohibit all types of moonlighting for his/her trainees. The Accreditation Committee for Graduate Medical Education (ACGME) has proposed that residents be allowed to work outside their training program only if their total combined educational program and moonlighting hours do not exceed the 80-hour weekly limits.

Reasons for Moonlighting

Many residents choose to work outside of residency for the extra income to supplement their residency stipend. The most common reasons for needing supplemental income are to support families and to repay medical school loans. The key benefits of moonlighting, besides the financial, are added clinical experience and an exposure to a patient population outside of the primary training program. External moonlighting also provides the opportunity for more autonomy in decision making in patient care.

Monitoring Moonlighting

The program director must ensure that moonlighting does not interfere with the ability of the resident to achieve the goals and objectives of the educational program. If a resident decides to moonlight, he may do so only with a written statement of permission from his or her program director. If a resident is not performing satisfactorily in the program, the program director may withdraw the permission to moonlight. The program director must comply with the sponsoring institution's written policies and procedures regarding moonlighting.

Requirements for External Moonlighting

You must first obtain a state medical license that allows for practice outside your training program, a controlled substance certificate from the state department of public health, and a personal federal DEA number to prescribe any schedule II drugs. Prior to starting work at many of the facilities, you will need to become a Medicare and Medicaid provider. Prior to accepting any moonlighting responsibilities, you must submit to your program director a letter listing the moonlighting activities, institutional affiliation, scope of the proposed activities, and the maximum number of hours (per week and per month) of proposed moonlighting.

Things to Look for Before Moonlighting

- *Internal moonlighting*: This is usually done in the emergency department, ICU, CCU and medical-surgical floor. One advantage is that you are already covered by the institution's liability insurance.
- *External moonlighting*: Residents often find opportunities in local hospitals that do not have training programs. These hospitals can usually provide you with malpractice insurance. Local school districts also need physicians to perform physical examinations for students wanting to participate in sports.
- *Work in large blocks of time*: Experienced residents suggest moonlighting when you have a lot of free time available. Try working through a free weekend or during a vacation to quickly earn a lump sum of cash.

Moonlighting Within Visa Regulations

In addition to the parameters outlined in this chapter, residents and fellows employed on a J-1, H-1B or O-1 visa are ineligible to moonlight, or have further restrictions, as follows:

- J-1 *Exchange Visitor*: No additional activity and/or compensation outside the defined parameters of the approved residency or fellowship training program is permitted.
- H-1B *Visitor*: Employment authorization is specific and limited to the position outlined in the employer's Labor Condition Application submitted to the Department of Labor (DoL) and the corresponding H-1B visa petition submitted to the U.S. Citizen and Immigration Service (USCIS). The employer may request

authorization for the foreign physician to train and perform services at multiple sites; however, all details must be included in the information submitted with the DoL application and visa petition. Employers who seek to amend the job description after the fact must follow specific DoL and USCIS reporting guidelines. Work or training opportunities (moonlighting) with a different employer require a separate DoL application and USCIS visa petition.

Medical Malpractice

Gerald P. Whelan and Vijay Rajput

IMGs coming to train and practice in the American medical system from other countries often have a great deal of concern about the issue of medical malpractice. Although it is probably true that physicians are taken to court and sued more often in the United States than in most other countries, by having good information about malpractice and following some basic principles of good medical practice, you can minimize the likelihood of becoming involved in a malpractice lawsuit.

The American legal system makes it relatively easy for a patient or family to initiate a malpractice lawsuit whenever they believe that the actions of a physician or hospital have resulted in wrongful injury or death. So the first point to realize is that being sued is not equivalent to being found guilty of malpractice. Although not absolutely required, most plaintiffs will engage an attorney to file the suit. Certain attorneys specialize in representing plaintiffs in a malpractice action, while others limit their practice to representing defendants.

There are several principles that you can follow in your practice that have been shown to minimize the likelihood of being sued. These include:

■ Patient-centered, evidence-based practice
■ Properly documented goals of care
■ Real-time communication with patient and families
■ Respect for patients' and families' input into patient-care decisions
■ Appropriate and timely disclosure of medical errors and unanticipated events
■ Sincere apologies for any errors or adverse outcomes

Although medical errors or incompetence may be a contributing factor in lawsuits, it is well documented that physicians who communicate poorly or have trouble establishing a rapport with their patients are far more likely to be sued or sanctioned by state medical boards.

You may hear your colleagues discussing "defensive medicine," the practice of ordering excessive or not-even-indicated laboratory and other studies to protect themselves from malpractice lawsuits. This has never been proven effective and only contributes to the spiraling cost of health care in the United States. The principles outlined above are the only defensive medicine that need be practiced.

What Constitutes Medical Malpractice?

There are four elements, all of which must be present for a physician or hospital to be guilty of medical malpractice. These include

1. The duty of a physician or hospital to treat the patient must be established.
2. There must be evidence of a breach of duty by the physician or hospital.
3. There must be evidence of injury caused directly by the breach of duty.
4. There must be damages that have occurred as a result of the injury.

In the event that you are involved in an adverse patient care outcome or death that may have been due to error or negligence or, in the case where the patient and/or family believes this to be true even if you feel there is no basis to their concern, there are several things you should do:

■ Immediately consult with your supervising resident and/or attending physician before meeting with the patient or family.
■ Immediately contact the risk management staff of your hospital.
■ Be sure that all medical records, laboratory results, images and other data are secure and accurate. However, never alter or attempt to change the medical record in any way!
■ After conferring with your supervisors and risk management staff, meet with the patient and/or family as soon as feasible. You may also defer this meeting to your senior residents or attending or have them accompany you.
■ Explain as clearly as possible, avoiding any medical jargon or equivocation, what has occurred and what the likely outcomes will be for the patient.
■ Allow the patient and/or family to ask questions and answer them as honestly as possible. Encourage them also to state their concerns about what has occurred.
■ Express appropriate and sincere sympathy for the adverse outcome or death but do not accept responsibility. Indicate that the case will be thoroughly investigated and no more information can be presented until that investigation is complete.

If the case goes forward you will likely have to give a sworn pre-trial deposition or appear in court to be questioned by attorneys. Both sets of attorneys will generally invoke testimony from expert witnesses, physicians with recognized expertise in the area under question but not directly involved in the case. Often the side with the most compelling expert witnesses wins the case. Understand that as a resident, you will be provided with malpractice insurance by your hospital when you sign your contract with your training program and, in reality, the ultimate legal responsibility for patient care lies with the attending physician. Nevertheless, even if you personally face no financial penalty, a finding against you can create problems with future insurance policies and hospital credentialing. For that reason, if you are involved in a case, take the matter very seriously and confer closely with the attorneys and risk managers which your hospital will provide for you.

In many cases a hospital may decide to settle the case "out of court". This means that a financial settlement is made with the plaintiff in return for dropping the charges.

Although this is probably better than being named in a suit that goes on to a finding of malpractice, it is not without consequence for your career. The hospital will make the final decision, but you are entitled to express your concerns, especially if you truly believe the suit is groundless.

MALPRACTICE INSURANCE

While malpractice insurance is provided by your hospital during your training, you will ultimately, as a practicing physician, have to buy your own malpractice insurance. The premium is based on the field of medicine, geographical location, and prior history of malpractice cases. There are some fields in medicine considered as having higher legal liability (e.g., gynecology and obstetrics, neurosurgery). This also depends upon the nature of practice (e.g., limiting practice to ambulatory gynecology).

If you are fully licensed in a state and still working as a resident or fellow but plan to work as an independent contractor (moonlighting), you need to make sure that you are covered by adequate insurance by the employing hospital or office. Because your residency program covers you for work only in your own institution, you need to protect yourself for services you perform outside your training program. Clinics and physician offices may offer additional malpractice insurance to moonlighters, but beware of coverage in the "claims-made" category. Claims-made insurance protects you from malpractice claims only if the insurer that covered you at the time of the alleged incident is the same as when the claim is actually filed. If that is not the case, you will not be covered unless you have purchased "tail insurance", which is designed to cover such after-the-fact claims. The only catch is that tail insurance can cost up to twice as much as standard malpractice insurance.

ACKNOWLEDGMENTS

My sincere thanks to Drs Ramaa Athreya, M. Attia, Carlos Rose, and M. Balasubramanian for sharing their experiences when they were newcomers to the U.S. health care system.—Balu Athreya

References

- **Accreditation Council for Graduate Medical Education.** Common program requirements. Link available at www.acgme.org/acWebsite/home/home.asp. Accessed 5 August 2008.
- **Athreya BH.** Clinical Competency Skills; 2006. Available at www.booklocker.com.
- **Girgis A, Sanson Fisher RW.** Breaking bad news: consensus guidelines for medical practitioners. J Clin Oncol. 1995;13:2449-56.
- **Kaboli PJ, Rosenthal GE.** Delays in transfer to ICU: a preventable adverse event? J Gen Intern Med. 2003;18:77-83.
- **Kluckhohn C.** Mirror for Man. Greenwich, CT: Fawcett Publications; 1967.
- **Sparrow M.** What it takes to be a senior resident. Hopkins Medical News. Fall 2001.
- **Spiegel JP.** Some cultural aspects of transference and counter-transference. In: Masserman JH, ed. Individual and Familial Dynamics. New York: Grune and Stratton; 1959:160-82.

8 Understanding the American Medical System

Edward Viner, MD, Ami Sharad Joshi, DO, MBA, Barbara A. Porter, MD, MPH, Vijay Rajput, MD, Patrick C. Alguire, MD, Susan K. Cavanaugh, MS, MPH, Nancy Calabretta, MS, MEd, Antoinette Spevetz, MD, Christy A. Rentmeester, PhD, Vani Dandolu, MD, MPH, and Gerald P. Whelan, MD

Typical Administrative Structure of Institution, Department, and Training Program — 135

Financial Issues Governing Resident Education: GME IME, and DME — 136

Medicare — 137

Medicaid — 138

Veterans Administration — 139

Emergency Medical Treatment and Active Labor Act (EMTALA) — 139

Public Health and Care of Uninsured — 139

Accreditation Council for Graduate Medical Education (ACGME) — 140

ACGME and Core Competency — 141

Duty Hours — 143

The Educational Process — 144

Education in the Clinical Environment — 144

- Supervised Direct Inpatient Care — 144
- Regularly Scheduled Didactic Sessions — 145

Residents as Teachers — 146

The Microskills Model (One-Minute Preceptor) — 147

- Get a Committment — 147
- Probe for Supporting Evidence — 148
- Teach General Rules — 148
- Reinforce What Was Done Right — 149
- Correct Mistakes — 149

Self-Directed Learning 150

Learning Resources: The Structure of the Medical Library 151

- Electronic and Print Resources 151

- The Medical Literature 152

- Managing References 153

- Critically Evaluating the Medical Literature 153

- Research Sponsored by Pharmaceutical Companies 155

- Simulation in Medical Education 156

Professionalism and Ethical Issues 158

- Confidentiality 158

- Informed Consent 159

- Respect, Autonomy, and Self-Determination 160

Learning within the Team System 161

- Graduated Levels of Responsibilities for Patient Care and Teaching 163

- Teaching Responsibilities 163

- Self-Study 165

Research Opportunities Before and During Residency 166

Before Residency: How Does Research Help IMGs? 166

How Do I Get Involved in a Research Project? 166

NIH, HRSA, and Private Industry 167

Academic Integrity and Scientific Integrity 167

- Research Misconduct 168

- Participation in Research During Residency 168

Typical Administrative Structure of Institution, Department, and Training Program

Edward Viner

Aall accredited training programs in the United States operate under the aegis of the Accreditation Council for Graduate Medical Education (ACGME) and must abide by its rules.

ACGME member organizations include the American Hospital Association, the American Board of Medical Specialties, the American Medical Association, the Association of American Medical Colleges and the Council of Medical Specialty Societies. Within the ACGME structure, there is a specific Residency Review Committee (RRC) for each specialty—for example, an RRC for internal medicine, another RRC for general surgery, and so on. There is also an RRC for each subspecialty fellowship program.

Every medical training program must have an organizational sponsor, which may be a medical school, a university or community hospital, or a free-standing outpatient clinic (in the latter case, such a clinic contracts with a hospital to provide the inpatient training component). This means that the administrative structure of graduate medical education is the same for all residency programs, no matter what type of sponsor.

Each sponsoring organization, in turn, has a Designated Institutional Official (DIO), who is responsible for administrative issues affecting all of the separate training programs offered by the organization. The DIO is usually, but not invariably, a physician. Generally, the DIO is responsible for contracts, salary structure, on-call rooms, human resource issues, policies and procedures, accreditation issues, grievances, and due process. Each training institution also must have a Committee of Graduate Medical Education, usually composed of the DIO, the department chiefs, program directors, and other personnel who are involved with the all of the institution's teaching programs. The ACGME is very specific about the structure, membership, and responsibilities of this committee.

The ACGME also dictates that each program must have adequate administrative support. Accordingly, most hospitals have an Office of Graduate Medical Education, headed by an individual who may be called the Director or Coordinator of Graduate Medical Education. This person reports to the DIO. In larger organizations, this office will also have other supporting staff, all of whom handle day-to-day administrative details for the residency programs. In addition, each of the institution's specific training programs will have a program director (PD), assistant program directors (APDs) and a coordinator. In programs that have IMGs on J-1 visas, there will also be an individual designated as the Training Program Liaison (TPL) who maintains contact between the IMG resident and ECFMG. All of these individuals may become very important to you on a personal basis.

The program director needs to ensure that the training program meets all of the RRC accreditation requirements (http://www.acgme.org). The program director is responsible for day-to-day program functions and reports to the departmental chair and DIO. The program coordinator is the person in charge of the day-to-day administrative activities of the program. He/she is a non-physician who helps in recruitment, orientation, documentation of evaluation, and other needs of the program and residents. In summary, the individuals with whom the trainee may interact include the DIO and staff, the PD and APDs, and the program coordinator, the TPL and the departmental teaching faculty. As already noted, the DIO is responsible for *institutional administrative issues* (e.g., if the on-call rooms are dirty, if your paycheck does not arrive). The PD and his or her assistants are responsible for the *content* of your program, guided by the rules and requirements of the program's specific RRC.

The role of a number of other individuals requires comment. Where the governing institution is a medical school, the top administrative officer is the dean. The dean influences GME through his/her appointment of the DIO, and via the department chairs who report to the dean. Where the sponsoring agent institution is a hospital, it is led by a president/chief executive officer who influences GME via the DIO, or the physician who is the hospital's chief medical officer.

The PD usually reports to the chairman/chief of the trainees' department, who in turn reports to the hospital's chief medical officer, and/or the medical school's dean, as the case may be. The department chair/chief is usually significantly involved in overseeing the training program and in creating the tone/culture of the department. However, this often is a largely behind-the-scenes role. In subspecialty programs, the division head is often the PD, although in large subspecialty divisions, the PD may be a division member who reports to the division head.

Last, but by no means least, the program's faculty usually is composed of a variable number of full-time physicians, who are salaried by the sponsoring institution, or by the medical school with which the hospital is associated. The faculty must be adequate in number and properly credentialed in their specialty to comply with the RRC rules. At many teaching hospitals, physicians in private practice also contribute importantly to the teaching program, on either a voluntary or a part-time salaried basis.

The other key people in the program are chief residents. The chief residents are the final-year residents in surgical programs or the third- or fourth-year residents in medicine, pediatrics, and emergency medicine programs. Chief residents plan the on-call duty assignments, educational conferences, and daily morning reports. Chief residents resolve conflicts between residents, manage administrative crises, manage the human resources (assign residents in case of sudden sick leave by residents etc.), and usually take on a significant teaching role.

In summary, it is the ACGME and its many RRCs that dictate the administrative structure to which the organizational sponsor must adhere, as well as the individual program's content and the extensive rules and regulations that DIOs and PDs must follow. A training program must be ACGME/RRC accredited for an institution to be eligible for reimbursement by the government for the cost of training residents, and trainees must successfully complete an accredited program in order to sit for specialty board certification examinations.

Financial Issues Governing Resident Education: GME, IME, and DME

Edward Viner

The sponsoring organization, which is most often a hospital, is reimbursed for residency training by the federal government through the Medicare program, which is the mechanism the government uses to pay for medical care for elderly and disabled individuals.

The money, which is collected through the income tax program, is used to reimburse hospitals for two separate components; the direct medical education costs (DME), which comprises trainees' salaries and fringe benefits, and the indirect medical education costs (IME), which includes the overhead costs incurred by the hospital by virtue of having a training program. The latter includes, among other things, the cost for on-call rooms, library, a portion of the program and assistant program directors' salaries, and those of the various support personnel.

The exact direct cost is determined by the annual cost report, provided by the institution to the federal government, accounting for expenses related to the training program. Hospitals get reimbursed for the direct cost of GME, based on the number of residents at the hospital at any one time, up to a specified maximum number for each hospital (the "cap"). This means that if the trainee is away on a month's elective at another institution, his "home program" does not get paid for that month because it cannot list that individual on its cost report for that period; yet, it must pay the trainee. Accordingly, this may affect your program's policy concerning away electives. On the other hand, if it is a regular and recurrent rotation, the "away" program may claim the trainees on its cost report, and therefore be reimbursed by the government. Then, by contractual agreement, the away institution can pay the home program, so the latter can recoup the cost of that individual's salary. While hospitals can legally exceed the number specified under the cap, the federal government will not pay for these extra positions. Accordingly, the cap practically limits the number of trainees a hospital can have at any one time.

Indirect costs are paid to training institutions based on a resident-to-bed count ratio. In some states, hospitals also get reimbursed for indirect overhead from the state's Medicaid program (which pays for the care of the poor). Nonetheless, the major source of funds for GME remains the federal government.

MEDICARE

Ami Sharad Joshi

Medicare was enacted by Congress in 1965 for financing the health care of the elderly. It has become the largest source of payment for medical services, primarily for the elderly, costing approximately $325 billion/year and 13% of the federal budget. Medicare is also the largest funding source for graduate medical education based on hospital-specific, per-resident amounts. Funding is based on the proportion of hospital days of patients who are accounted as Medicare patients and the number of full-time residents training in the hospital. The majority of these funds are collected through payroll taxation of the general population, partially through the Federal Insurance Contributions Act and Self Employment Contributions Act. Individuals who are eligible for Medicare must be U.S. citizens or permanent legal residents for five continuous years and more than 65 years of age. Other eligible individuals include those who are younger than age 65 but who are disabled and have received Social Security for more than two years, those with end-stage renal disease on dialysis, and those with amyotrophic lateral sclerosis.

There are two major parts to Medicare: Part A for hospital services and Part B for physician services, nursing services, laboratory tests, diagnostic tests, and outpatient hospital procedures. Eligible beneficiaries are automatically enrolled in part A, whereas enrollment in Part B is voluntary and requires payment of an insurance premium. In 2006, Congress enacted Medicare Part D to help with prescription coverage because Medicare beneficiaries were found to have inadequate coverage for their prescription medications. Medicare

Part D allows beneficiaries to participate in drug plans by traditional insurers or others (i.e., patients are eligible to add an additional prescription drug plan to cover what traditional Medicare does not).

As for physicians, payments are based on a Medicare physician fee schedule. Each physician is first given a unique physician number (UPIN) that identifies them for Medicare payments and services. The Centers for Medicare and Medicaid Services then developed a formula to pay practice services for those who see Medicare patients. This formula is based on total practice expenses and resources required for individual services. The payment has to be adequate enough to encourage physicians to see Medicare beneficiaries, but at the same time not waste Medicare's scant resources. Medicare physician payment is determined by the Medicare Fee Schedule, and Congress assists in calculating annual spending. If annual physician spending exceeds target goals, then reimbursement rates are decreased. Because of these discrepancies in payments, value-based purchasing has been initiated as a way to reward practices for providing better quality care (i.e., paying for high-quality efficient patient care based on practices using evidence that informs critical decision making). As a result, the Department of Health and Human Services Agency for Healthcare and Research Quality published quality indicator measurements to help assess patient care. Included in those indicators are prevention services, inpatient quality measures, and patient safety markers, which can be used to create a performance report on hospitals and practices. The government hopes that this will avoid duplicate services, eliminate unnecessary services, encourage preventive health, and adequately compensate physician services.

MEDICAID

Ami Sharad Joshi

Medicaid was established in 1965 through Title XIX of the Social Security Act to provide financial health care assistance to mothers, the aged, the blind, and the disabled. It is a joint federal–state program that provides health insurance to low-income individuals, children, disabled patients, and pregnant women who are eligible. Poverty alone does not qualify a person to receive benefits. In addition, because each state runs its own program, eligibility varies from state to state. Eligibility is based on two basic criteria: financial needs and federally recognized eligibility (disability, dependent children in a household). Unlike private insurers, Medicaid cannot exclude individuals based on pre-existing illnesses or limit services without meeting specific criteria.

Medicaid has expanded its coverage to a large proportion of patients with HIV/AIDS, babies and children, pregnant women, and elderly and disabled persons who meet pre-defined eligibility requirements. In 2002, Medicaid enrolled 39.9 million Americans and 18.4 million were children. Medicaid also aids in funding more than half of nursing home expenditures, and supports teaching institutions, migrant health centers, and psychiatric hospitals.

Medicaid is funded through the state with a matching federal program based on a state's per capita income, utilizing an average of 22% of each state's budget. The wealthiest state receives a federal match of 50%; poorer states receive a greater amount. Unfortunately, with a growing population and an increasing number of beneficiaries, Medicaid state expenses are increasing. As a result, states are trying to reduce their Medicaid expenditures by controlling prescription drug costs, restricting eligibility, increasing co-payments for the members, and reducing benefits.

VETERANS ADMINISTRATION

Ami Sharad Joshi

The United States Department of Veteran Affairs provides medical benefits for all enrolled veterans. This plan provides outpatient and inpatient services within the Veterans Administration (VA) health care system. Those that are eligible include active military service agents and the honorably discharged. Services include preventive care services (immunizations, physical exams, and health education programs), outpatient diagnostic and treatment services, surgical, mental health, emergency department services, and inpatient treatment.

The VA health care system has adopted primary care as its foundation by aligning human resources to primary care, implementing primary case-based quality-improvement programs, and developing electronic medical records to enhance communication, scheduling and physician order entry. The VA system emphasizes coordinated continuous care, from primary to specialist, including over 1200 facilities, 770 ambulatory clinics, 170 hospitals, and 132 nursing homes. Over one-third of resident physicians spend time in the VA health care system (see the article by Stevens, Holland, and Kizer in the Reference section at the end of this chapter).

To increase medical service to the VA system, President Clinton enacted the Nursing Relief for Disadvantaged Areas Act of 1999, which allowed immigrants to practice in the VA system and underserved areas in order to fulfill their national interest waver criteria and ultimately obtain permanent residents status. Immigrants with J-1 visas can work within this system and provide overall health care for the underserved.

EMERGENCY MEDICAL TREATMENT AND ACTIVE LABOR ACT (EMTALA)

Ami Sharad Joshi

In 1986, the Emergency Medical Treatment and Active Labor Act (EMTALA) was enacted to prevent 'patient dumping'. This act prevented emergency departments from refusing care to the indigent and uninsured by transferring them to other institutions. It requires all emergency departments that participate in Medicare to provide a medical exam and treatment to all patients regardless of their ability to pay. Hospitals must also maintain specialists on-call for the emergency department. If the hospital is unable to stabilize the patient, they are required to transfer the patient to the appropriate center for care. Follow-up care is also to be arranged for patients who need outpatient services. Hospitals not regulated by EMTALA include military, VA hospitals, Indian Health Services, and Shriner Hospitals for children.

EMTALA has led to positive and negative consequences. It is beneficial in that all people have access to emergency services, but as a result more than half of emergency care goes uncompensated and many hospitals have been forced to close their emergency departments.

PUBLIC HEALTH AND CARE OF UNINSURED

Ami Sharad Joshi

The proportion of the United States population without insurance is higher than it was 20 years ago. The uninsured include the unemployed and their families, employees whose employers do not offer health insurance, and those who are self-employed and have not purchased health insurance. The biggest increase in the uninsured is in the working adult population (i.e., 18 to 64 years of age). In addition, young adults and Hispanics were found to be the least likely to have health insurance. In 2005, 45.8 million Americans were uninsured, while 16 million of the insured are actually underinsured and not receiving adequate medical coverage. Unfortunately, those who are uninsured often end up with medical disorders that are diagnosed late in their course, have access to fewer preventive care services, and ultimately have worse health care outcomes. Because the uninsured have worse health outcomes than the insured, the cost of their care is greater, creating a financial burden for the government that is ultimately borne by the taxpayer.

Within each community, there exists a "safety net" health care system for the uninsured. The safety net varies from state to state depending on the marketplace, Medicaid reimbursements, and state financial support. In some areas the state and/or county provide uncompensated hospital and emergency care, whereas in other jurisdictions public and privately owned systems provide care to the uninsured. States where there are more uninsured people (Texas, California, and Florida) have higher financial stresses related to the provision of medical care.

The real challenge now lies in making insurance coverage affordable to the uninsured. A few states are pioneering a solution for a trend towards universal coverage. Some of the program elements include high-deductible coverage, financial reward for preventive care, and penalties for failure to comply with treatment. In addition, this new plan will focus on individuals' obligations to their own health care, and at the same time the government will protect individuals' insurance plans during economic/social change. This strategy responds to the growing concern for American working persons who are uninsured.

Charity care is free or at a reduced charge to patients who receive services at an acute care hospital. In New Jersey, for example, charity care provides health care reimbursements to patients who lack private health insurance and whose income falls below a set amount but is too high to qualify for Medicaid. Charity care may not include anesthesiology fees, radiology, and outpatient prescriptions.

Accreditation Council for Graduate Medical Education (ACGME)

Ami Sharad Joshi

The Accreditation Council for Graduate Medical Education (ACGME) is an organization that was established in 1981 to evaluate and accredit graduate medical education programs in the United States. The purpose of this body is to enhance graduate medical education for residents and fellows and at the same time improve the quality of health care provided in the United States. The ACGME establishes policies for graduate medical education institutions. During the academic year of 2006-2007, there were 8502 ACGME-accredited residency and fellowship programs in 120 specialties and subspecialties and 104,879 residents and fellows in supervised GME programs. The ACGME consists of 28 committees, which include specialty committees, a committee for a 1-year transitional year residency and hospital/institutional committees. Each committee is composed of 6 to 15 volunteer physician members including resident representatives.

The bulk of the ACGME work is done by its Residency Review Committees (RRC), national committees representing each of 26 medical specialties and consisting of faculty and resident members. RRC members are appointed by the AMA Council on Medical Education and by specialty boards and organizations. These committees establish (subject to ACGME approval) special requirements for each medical specialty and evaluate residency programs against these standards. The RRC evaluates residency programs directly via site surveys and review of documents. Site surveyors formally interview residents and faculty in the program and evaluate the documentation of the program's compliance with RRC and ACGME requirements. Programs typically are accredited for 3 to 5 years. The program may be placed on probation or be terminated if they do not meet established standards. Programs that are on probation have a responsibility to inform applicants and residents of their status, and programs that are terminated (a rare event) have a responsibility to assist residents in finding positions in other programs. The RRC's ultimate goal is to ensure a proper balance between service and education during the residency.

ACGME AND CORE COMPETENCY

Over the past several years, ACGME, the Council on Graduate Medical Education, the AAMC, the Federal Council on Internal Medicine, and other groups began to recognize the growing need for a change in the education of physicians in training. As a result, the ACGME reviewed the current process of graduate medical education and focused on the outcomes of education and the competencies needed by physicians of the future. The ACGME employed the Dreyfus Model of Knowledge (Table 8-1) to model an educational process for physicians to grow from competency to proficiency.

TABLE 8-1

Dreyfus Model of Skill Acquisition

Level	Description
Novice	Needs to be told exactly what to do; has very little context to make decisions or plan management. The stage is represented by first-year medical students developing history and physical examination skills.
Advanced beginner	Has more context for decision making but still follows rigid guidelines. This stage is characterized by the junior medical student who manages hospitalized patients under the supervision of a resident or attending.
Competent	Begins to question the reasoning behind the tasks and can see longer-term consequences. This stage includes the first-year resident learning how to manage patients.
Proficient	Still relies on rules but is able to separate what is most important. This stage is characteristic of the newly practicing physician.

In addition, the ACGME in conjunction with other groups, including the ABMS, identified six Core Competencies (Table 8-2) which encompassed specific skills, knowledge, behavior, and learning opportunities for physicians in training. Programs are held accountable for teaching and evaluating the competencies by their respective RRCs.

The first core competency is Patient Care. Within this competency, residents are evaluated on their knowledge and skills with respect to medical history and physical examination, differential diagnosis, therapeutic interventions, patient counseling, patient

TABLE 8-2

ACGME Core Competencies*

Patient Care

Residents must be able to provide patient care that is compassionate, appropriate, and effective for the treatment of health problems and the promotion of health. Residents are expected to:
- Communicate effectively and demonstrate caring and respectful behaviors when interacting with patients and their families
- Gather essential and accurate information about their patients
- Make informed decisions about diagnostic and therapeutic interventions based on patient information and preferences, up-to-date scientific evidence, and clinical judgment
- Develop and carry out patient management plan
- Counsel and educate patients and their families
- Use information technology to support patient care decisions and patient education
- Perform competently all medical and invasive procedures considered essential for the area of practice
- Provide health care services aimed at preventing health problems or maintaining health
- Work with health care professionals, including those from other disciplines, to provide patient-focused care

Medical Knowledge

Residents must demonstrate knowledge about established and evolving biomedical, clinical, and cognate (e.g., epidemiological and social-behavioral) sciences and the application of this knowledge to patient care. Residents are expected to:
- Demonstrate an investigatory and analytic thinking approach to clinical situations
- Know and apply the basic and clinically supportive sciences that are appropriate to their discipline

Practice-Based Learning and Improvement

Residents must be able to investigate and evaluate their patient care practices, appraise and assimilate scientific evidence, and improve their patient care practices. Residents are expected to:
- Analyze practice experience and perform practice-based improvement activities using a systematic methodology
- Locate, appraise, and assimilate evidence from scientific studies related to their patients' health problem(s)
- Obtain and use information about their own population of patients and the larger population from which their patients are drawn
- Apply knowledge of study designs and statistical methods to the appraisal of clinical studies and other information on diagnostic and therapeutic effectiveness
- Use information technology to manage information, access on-line medical information, and support their own education
- Facilitate the learning of students and other health care professionals

Interpersonal and Communication Skills

Residents must be able to demonstrate interpersonal and communication skills that result in effective information exchange and teaming with patients, their patients' families, and professional associates. Residents are expected to:
- Create and sustain a therapeutic and ethically sound relationship with patients
- Use effective listening skills and elicit and provide information using effective nonverbal, explanatory, questioning, and writing skills
- Work effectively with others as a member or leader of a health care team or other professional group

Professionalism

Residents must demonstrate a commitment to carrying out professional responsibilities, adherence to ethical principles, and sensitivity to a diverse patient population. Residents are expected to:
- Demonstrate respect, compassion, and integrity; a responsiveness to the needs of patients and society that supercedes self-interest; accountability to patients, society, and the profession; and a commitment to excellence and on-going professional development
- Demonstrate a commitment to ethical principles pertaining to provision or withholding of clinical care, confidentiality of patient information, informed consent, and business practices
- Demonstrate sensitivity and responsiveness to patients' culture, age, gender, and disabilities

Systems-Based Practice

Residents must demonstrate an awareness of and responsiveness to the larger context and system of health care and the ability to effectively call on system resources to provide care that is of optimal value. Residents are expected to:
- Understand how their patient care and other professional practices affect other health care professionals, the health care organization, and the larger society and how these elements of the system affect their own practice
- Know how types of medical practice and delivery systems differ from one another, including methods of controlling health care costs and allocating resources
- Practice cost-effective health care and resource allocation that does not compromise quality of care
- Advocate for quality patient care and assist patients in dealing with system complexities
- Know how to partner with health care managers and health care providers to assess, coordinate, and improve health care and know how these activities can affect system performance

*For an electronic version of this table, see http://www.acgme.org/outcome/comp/compHome.asp. Used with permission of the Accreditation Counsel for Graduate Medical Education. Copyright © 2003 by ACGME.

management, and discharge planning. The second competency of Medical Knowledge evaluates residents on their problem-solving skills, analytic abilities, and use of current evidenced-based medical knowledge. Practice-Based Learning and Improvement is the third competency and encourages residents to identify areas of potential improvement in patient care practices and then use scientific methods to implement strategies to improve deficiencies. Under the fourth core competency, a resident is assessed for his/her written and verbal Interpersonal and Communication Skills with patients and colleagues. The fifth core competency evaluates a resident's skills as a Professional, including respectful and ethical behavior towards patients and co-workers and recognizing and acknowledging patient diversity. This competency also addresses patient confidentiality. The last core competency is System-Based Practice, which is the ability to identify specific areas of potential improvement within the process of health care delivery. Residents are expected to improve patient safety and treatment through overall system improvement. This may entail identification of medical errors related to the process of care and developing systemic solutions.

DUTY HOURS

The Accreditation Council for Graduate Medical Education implemented duty-hour requirements for all residency programs in June 2002 to promote patient safety and resident well-being and to shift the focus away from resident service to resident education. These regulations were put in place for three reasons: 1) better management of an increasing patient population with greater severity of illness, 2) public opinion that long hours compromise patient safety, and 3) research showing that sleep deprivation affects resident performance. Interestingly, Europe and Australia had already implemented duty hours for *all* hospital workers at 48-56 hours/week. Duty hours are defined as the number of hours a resident may participate in activities in a hospital or ambulatory clinic, including both clinical and academic activities (e.g., patient care, administrative duties related to patient care, conferences). Excluded in these hours are reading and other hospital preparation time spent outside the hospital. These limits were designed to enhance resident well-being, prevent fatigue and sleep deprivation and, most importantly, to prevent any negative effects on patient care and learning.

The specifics of duty hours are as follows:

■ No resident shall work greater than an average of 80 hours per week over a 4-week period, including moonlighting hours. An exception may be granted to programs for a maximum of 88 hours if they can deliver a sound, educational reason to the ACGME and the ACGME approves. (Before implementation of these restrictions, residents were working an average of 100 hours/week, and 36-48 hours consecutively.)
■ Residents will have 1 in 7 days off from the hospital, including all educational activities.
■ In-hospital call will be no more frequent than every third night and, when a resident is on call, he or she will not accept new patient care after 24 hours on call.
■ Residents will remain in the hospital for no more than 6 hours following their 24-hour call. Following their in-house call, residents will have a minimum of 10-hour off time for themselves before the beginning of their next hospital activity. For at-home call, the same rules are not applicable except for the 1 day in 7; that

one day is to be completely free for the resident from hospital activities. However, residents are not to be on call so frequently as to hinder the resident's rest and safety.

The Educational Process

The medical educational process is focused on and directly involves patients and their problems. This direct care of the patient lies at the heart of medical education. In the United States, undergraduate medical schools provide substantial clinical exposure during clerkships and sub-internships, usually during the third and fourth years of medical school. During residency and fellowship training, known as graduate medical education (GME), "on the job" clinical education is the core of professional and academic development. The ultimate goal of GME is to transcend simply enabling residents to achieve passing scores on board examinations and meet licensure requirements, and ensure that residents are transformed into effective and efficient physicians who deliver the best patient care possible.

Education in the clinical environment is a challenge for the teacher as well as for residents. The ACGME and individual RRCs mandate where and how clinical and didactic education is to be provided to residents. Almost all doctors trained in the United States are involved in teaching at some point in their career. Most undertake the job conscientiously and passionately; however, very few receive formal training in teaching skills. In the past it was presumed that if you know the subject well, you can teach well, although in reality this is not necessarily true. Many teaching programs now provide a faculty development course for their faculty who teach, which instructs teachers in some of the basic tenets of medical education. Resident education occurs through a constellation of large group seminars, small group or individualized tutorials, and through "on the job" teaching in the patient care setting. Residents learn not just from faculty, but from near-peers such as students and resident colleagues.

In this section, we describe the various types of clinical teaching and identify common educational challenges in the clinical environment, describing how these can affect the IMG entering a U.S. residency program.

EDUCATION IN THE CLINICAL ENVIRONMENT

Barbara A. Porter and Vijay Rajput

Supervised Direct Inpatient Care

Typically, residents care for hospitalized patients admitted to a teaching attending physician. Many hospitals also have parallel non-teaching services, where residents are not involved in patient care. Patients are usually admitted from emergency departments, but also come from outpatient offices like urgent care clinics, resident outpatient clinics, or private physicians' offices. The majority of inpatients in the United States are admitted emergently, not electively.

In most residencies, the majority of patient care is managed by a resident team, composed of the first-year resident, (often called the "intern") and supervised by a senior resident. Overall responsibility and supervision falls on an attending physician. The team may also include medical students or other students from health-related fields and may include more than just two residents.

Upon a patient's admission to the hospital, the senior resident supervises the history and physical examination, assessment, and plan developed and documented by the first-year resident. On the day of admission, the patient's presentation is reviewed with the attending physician as well, who helps guide the team in the care of the patient. Likewise, the daily work of patient care is performed by the resident team, with ultimate supervision and responsibility provided by the attending physician.

In most disciplines and programs, there are two types of daily patient care rounds: work rounds and attending teaching rounds. Generally, work rounds are directed by the senior resident with the goal of teaching and learning the fundamental skills for caring for hospitalized patients, while getting the daily patient care work completed (e.g., interpreting data, placing orders, calling consultants). Attending teaching rounds are rounds directed by the attending physician, and entail formal presentations of patient cases by the students and residents, with discussion by the attending physician. Often the attending physician will model physical exam and communication skills to the team or observe team members demonstrating these skills. Sometimes attending teaching rounds will mimic work rounds and include higher level teaching about management, and may incorporate nonmedical issues such as resource utilization.

Regularly Scheduled Didactic Sessions

Didactic education remains a significant component of residency education in the United States. While the format of education varies between disciplines and institutions, there is usually a variety of didactic sessions at every program. Below are some commonly occurring didactic sessions.

Morning report is a traditional daily meeting in internal medicine and pediatric residency programs. It is a core teaching conference where discussion of patient care and exchange of information is emphasized. Morning report has different formats, but usually there is a presentation of one or two cases by residents, with chief residents or faculty leading the discussion. Morning report is usually attended by all residents and medical students on inpatient services.

Teaching attending rounds are mandated by the ACGME to occur a minimum of three days per week, for a minimum resident contact time of 4.5 hours per week. Residents present cases and demonstrate clinical skills at the bedside. This "conference" assimilates basic science knowledge, clinical data, pathophysiology, and evidence-based principles related to the patient and allows for critical feedback of resident decision making. The bedside component includes assessment of the residents' history, physical examination, and communication skills, and allows for modeling by the teaching attending physician.

Chairman's rounds are a weekly conference conducted by the chairman of the department. The format of this conference varies by institution and may be bedside rounds with the chairman and a small group of residents or a case-based conference where the discussion is facilitated by the chairman.

Grand rounds is a weekly scholarly presentation by local or visiting faculty, which is attended by students, residents and faculty.

Journal club is an ACGME-mandated conference conducted at least monthly. Usually an article from current medical literature is discussed, with lessons on critical reading of the medical literature and evidence-based medicine.

The *morbidity and mortality* (M&M) *conference* is conducted by residents and faculty as part of their scholarly activity and in most institutions occurs monthly. Traditionally, M&M conferences were based on sentinel events (i.e., medical error or an unexpected poor outcome) occurring in the hospital. Typically the case in question is presented by a resident, and the faculty and residents discuss the case with the goal of learning from medical error. There is a movement away from the traditional "blame and shame" culture of M&M to a more proactive stance towards patient safety and quality and system improvement. Similar to M&M is the autopsy conference. A case is presented and the autopsy report is then discussed, including a review of pathological specimens.

The *core curriculum conference* consists of a series of didactic lectures of fundamental clinical and scientific topics pertinent to each specialty, as well as special topics addressing the ACGME core competencies. Topics are repeated in 12-18-month cycles to ensure adequate opportunity for all residents to attend core conferences. Depending on the institution, these core lectures are offered as a half-day session per week or as daily noon conferences.

Some residency programs offer *board review conferences* as part of their didactic series. A board review "course" is a set of conferences focused on preparation for the American Board of Medical Specialties examinations. Some programs offer board review on a weekly basis, where practice questions are reviewed and a faculty facilitator discusses the question, provides a critique for the correct answer, and responds to resident questions.

Many programs begin the intern year with a series of conferences intended specifically for interns to review management of commonly encountered medical problems.

RESIDENTS AS TEACHERS

Patrick C. Alguire

Many programs offer conferences that help residents develop teaching and leadership skills. These conferences are often offered at the end of intern year to help prepare interns for their transition to a supervising and teaching resident.

In practice, a great deal of the teaching in GME programs is provided by residents who teach those more junior to them. Chief residents teach senior residents who in turn teach junior residents who in turn teach medical students. This "near peer" teaching has the added advantage of the teacher still being aware of the limits of knowledge of the learner because they were in the same position only the year before. Hence, a few tips on clinical teaching may be helpful.

The traditional model of case-based learning is familiar to residents. A learner presents a case and you must then create educational opportunities for the learner that relate to the case and provide care for the patient. These tasks might be accomplished by

- Role modeling ("Watch me care for the patient.")
- Questioning ("Tell me what you think and why.")
- Performing expert consultation ("Ask me what you need to know.")
- Mini-lecturing ("I will tell you what I know about this topic.")
- Modeling problem solving ("I will think out loud about this case.")
- Encouraging self-directed, independent learning ("What do you need to read about to understand this case?")
- Assigning teacher-directed, independent learning ("I think you should look this up.")

Most teachers use a combination of techniques, and, with experience, preceptors learn to choose which model is right for a specific situation.

THE MICROSKILLS MODEL (ONE-MINUTE PRECEPTOR)

Patrick C. Alguire

Nether and coworkers have broken down case-based teaching into five Microskills that facilitate learning. This method uses the technique of questioning to understand and address learner and patient needs efficiently and effectively. It allows you 1) to assess what the learner does and does not know, 2) to instruct the learner, and 3) to provide feedback more efficiently. This teaching model can be easily learned and is modestly associated with improved ratings of teaching skills. The Microskills model is associated with more teaching about the patient's specific illness including differential diagnosis, testing, and disease presentation. Teachers who use the Microskills have improved confidence in their feedback skills, and give more specific feedback to learners. Finally, teachers trained in the Microskills model spent more time listening to the presentation and soliciting understanding of the learners' thinking and less time eliciting data from the learner.

Microskills can be used with nearly any level of learner skill. The five rules are listed below.

1. Get a commitment. ("What do you think is going on with this patient?")
2. Probe for supporting evidence. ("Why do you think that?")
3. Teach general rules. ("Always do this when you see a similar case.")
4. Reinforce what was done right. ("Here is what you did right, and this is why it is important.")
5. Correct mistakes. ("I will tell you what you can do better; I will tell you how to do it better.")

Get a Commitment

The first Microskill asks the learner to commit to some decision or plan of action (Box 8-1). The cue to use this Microskill is when the learner pauses after presenting a patient, waiting for you to offer an explanation of the findings or a course of action. At this point, instead of taking over the case and solving the problem and inadvertently missing a teaching opportunity, you should ask, "What do you think is going on?" Other appropriate questions might include, "What do you want to do" or "How would you manage this?" Asking for a commitment encourages the learner to feel more responsible for the patient,

---

☑ **BOX 8-1   Getting a Commitment**

Helpful Approaches
- "What do you think is going on with this patient?"
- "Why do you think the patient continues to be hypertensive on three medications?"
- "What do you want to accomplish during this visit?"

These questions are characterized by expecting the learner to offer explanations, not just "yes" or "no" answers; the learner must elaborate upon his or her knowledge.

Unhelpful Approaches
- "Sounds like pneumonia, don't you think?"
- "Did you consider CHF as the cause of the dyspnea?"

These questions do not demand elaboration of knowledge by the learner; they can be answered "yes" or "no", and the answer is often prompted by the nature of the question.

forces active learning, and engenders a sense of collaboration with you. Learners who make mistakes reveal gaps in their knowledge or judgment that can be addressed by you, either with a short explanation or with a follow-up reading assignment.

Probe for Supporting Evidence

After you get the learner to make a commitment, ask the learner for the evidence that supports the commitment. Instead of saying, "You are right" or "You are wrong," ask questions like "What were the major findings that led you to that diagnosis?" or "Why did you choose furosemide rather than hydrochlorothiazide?" Questions help the learner reflect on the mental steps that were used to make the commitment. It is important to remember that probing for more information is not the same as "grilling" learners, and it helps to emphasize to the learner that this is a process to help them "think out loud." It also gives you a chance to analyze a learner's diagnostic abilities by understanding how the learner came to his or her conclusion. The core of this model is to first diagnose the learner. These first two steps are essential to doing this. They help you find out what the learner is thinking and avoids a situation where the learner is trying to guess what you want to hear (Box 8-2).

☑ BOX 8-2   Probing for Supporting Evidence

Helpful Approaches
- "What about his presentation led you to this diagnosis?"
- "How did you decide that Mrs Smith has pneumonia?"
- "What did you find on exam that makes you think this is a surgical abdomen?"
- "What were the factors that made you consider esophageal reflux rather than cardiac ischemia?"

These questions are characterized by asking the learner to demonstrate his or her thinking as it pertains to the case at hand. The learner must synthesize collected data and content knowledge to justify the diagnosis.

Unhelpful Approaches
- "What are the possible causes of dyspnea on exertion?"
- "I don't think this is PID. Do you have any other ideas?"
- "This seems like a clear case of gout to me; how about you?"
- "What are the five most common bacterial causes of community-acquired pneumonia?"

These questions are characterized by either having the learner create lists of diagnoses that may not be pertinent to the patient's problem or are leading questions that do not permit thoughtful consideration of the problem.

Questions coupled with immediate feedback are powerful teaching tools that, with practice, can be mastered by any preceptor. These questions also make excellent evaluation tools. When used sequentially, they allow you to assess the skill level of the learner—that is, is the learner capable of only reporting the data or can he or she synthesize, justify, and demonstrate good judgment and decision-making skills?

Teach General Rules

Whenever possible, attempt to teach a general rule (Box 8-3). General rules represent teaching scripts or "pearls" that are often presented effortlessly as they represent learning points gleaned from clinical experience. They commonly can be presented in one or two sentences. When something is offered as a general rule, it is more memorable and easily transferable to other cases than if offered as a patient-specific plan. Importantly, it is not imperative to "teach" something with each patient encounter. If the learner has done well, give positive feedback and save the formal teaching for another case.

☑ **BOX 8-3** **Teaching General Rules**

Helpful Approaches
- "If a young adult has mechanical low-back pain, x-rays are usually not helpful."
- "It is helpful to address code status while patients are still healthy so that you can have a meaningful discussion."
- "When following up a case of pneumonia, remember that the infiltrates on the chest x-ray might not clear for 4 to 6 weeks. It is best to postpone the follow-up x-ray until after that time."

These approaches are characterized by creating "rules of thumb" that can be applied reasonably to similar cases. They are short and to the point. The learner can be challenged to look up the scientific rationale for these rules as an independent learning assignment.

Unhelpful Approaches
- "Mr. Smith does not need a back x-ray today."
- "Why don't we discuss code status with Mrs Jones today?"
- "Arrange for Mr. Doe to have his repeat chest x-ray at the end of the month."
- "I always treat pneumonia with two antibiotics because patients seem to do better."
- "I never give a flu and pneumonia vaccination at the same time. It might make the patient sick."

These approaches address a specific, rather than a general, problem. They may also represent an unsupported, idiosyncratic approach to patient care. It often takes an insightful physician to recognize and correct this approach.

Reinforce What Was Done Right

This is sometimes referred to as "catching the learner doing something well." When the learner does well, reinforce what was done correctly by providing positive and specific feedback. Even learners who are doing well may not recognize which elements of their behavior are helpful and, thus, which behaviors to continue. Positive feedback helps promote self-esteem and builds confidence and probably heightens awareness to corrective criticism when it is offered. Positive feedback should not be mistaken for general praise ("You did a good job with that last patient") but should be explicit, reinforcing desired behaviors. Effective positive feedback also includes a probable outcome of the observed behavior and provides a rationale for continuing it. For example, "You were very empathic with that patient, and she responded by providing important information in the history" (Box 8-4).

☑ **BOX 8-4** **Reinforcing What Was Done Right**

Helpful Approaches
- "You evaluated this in a stepwise fashion and considered the patient's preferences in your suggestions. As a result, she is likely to be compliant with our recommendations."
- "You did a good job noting the possible role of medication side effects in the diagnosis. This helped us avoid unnecessary tests."

These statements are characterized by providing specific praise that targets a specific action or behavior and the associated real or potential outcome of that action or behavior.

Unhelpful Approaches
- "Strong work!"
- "You did a great job on that last case."

General praise that does not specify the precise action or behavior that was helpful (or how it was likely to be helpful) characterizes unhelpful feedback. The learner will not know exactly what was good, why it was good, or how to duplicate it.

Correct Mistakes

Learners make mistakes; when they do, supply corrective feedback. Remember that learners rarely make mistakes on purpose; most errors that persist are the result of insufficient feedback. For the feedback to be effective, you must choose an appropriate time and place to present the criticism to the learner. It is useful to begin by having learners review their own performance. Most learners have remarkable insight into their weaknesses and tend to be harder on themselves than their supervisors. Follow up the learner's comments with your own observations. Attempt to frame the observation of the mistake as "not the best" rather than "bad" or "wrong." Then, provide specific guidance on improvement, for example, by saying "You may be more successful next time this happens if you try..." and by giving them an opportunity to practice (Box 8-5).

☑ BOX 8-5　Correcting Mistakes

Helpful Approaches
- "I agree that Goodpasture's is a possible diagnosis, but bacterial sinusitis is much more likely based on disease prevalence and lack of other findings. Next time, consider common conditions first."
- "Your diagnosis is correct, but she cannot afford the medication you recommended. Next time consider the patient's financial circumstances when recommending medications."
This feedback is characterized by identifying a specific behavior or action that needs correction and what needs to be done to improve the next time.

Unhelpful Approaches
- "You actually ordered that?"
- "I can't believe you know so little for a fourth-year student."
These statements are vague or judgmental and are not accompanied with advice on how to improve. Avoid these kinds of statements!

What makes this model so appealing to both teachers and learners is that it de-emphasizes the effect of transferring "new knowledge" and showcases everyday patient-management skills.

SELF-DIRECTED LEARNING

Patrick C. Alguire

It may seem that you have more opportunities for learning than you have time for as a resident. One of the most significant skills you should develop as a resident is the skill of self-directed learning. Self-directed learning requires discipline. Self-directed learning occurs when you read about the patient you are caring for, when you ask questions of your consultants, and when you research the literature about a vexing problem. In fact, it is your self-directed learning skill set that will keep you current as a physician, long after residency is over.

The two essential steps in self-directed learning are the identification of the limits of one's knowledge and skills and the ability to organize resources to learn more. To maximize effectiveness, self-directed learning should be linked to a recently observed patient problem. Box 8-6 summarizes the main components of self-directed learning.

☑ BOX 8-6　Main Components of Self-Directed Learning

- Identify the Learning Need
  After a case presentation, identify your learning question by asking yourself, "What bothers me most about this case?"
- Give Yourself an Assignment
  Formulate the learning question, then research it.
- Identify Resources
  Potential resources include textbooks, journals, consultants, and PubMed and other electronic databases.
- "Close the Loop"
  Report back to the team or incorporate your newly found knowledge in a patient write-up or assessment.

LEARNING RESOURCES: THE STRUCTURE OF THE MEDICAL LIBRARY

Susan K. Cavanaugh and Nancy Calabretta

Medical libraries vary in size, services, and resources based on the institutions they are designed to support. These libraries range from a multi-story, well-funded academic medical center facility to a small, one-person library with minimal resources. Larger libraries employ library support staff as well as librarians. Support staff provide services such as circulation of materials, inter-library loan, and photocopying. Librarians manage library services, select resources, and provide reference services such as research and training. All libraries require users to register in order to borrow print materials and to have access to electronic resources paid for by the institution. These resources are available only to faculty, staff and students of the institution and require a password-protected login. Check with library staff before making multiple copies from any resource in order to avoid copyright violations. They can also offer guidance in the policies regarding computer use within your institution.

Get to know the librarians. They are experts with graduate degrees in information science and can help you perform information searches. They can save you time by answering your questions, teaching you how to search, and doing searches to find what you haven't been able to find on your own. Ask the librarians to provide an overview of the resources and services available. They are also invaluable in directing you to authoritative Web sites from specialty societies (e.g., ACP), government agencies (e.g., NIH), and non-governmental health care organizations (e.g., American Heart Association).

Electronic and Print Resources

Library Web Page
■ Gateway to library resources
■ Most libraries require users to access resources that the library pays for through the Web page

Online Catalog
■ Check holdings, locations, and formats

Databases
■ Free databases (e.g., PubMed)
■ Subscription databases (e.g., Cochrane Library, Westlaw)

Books/CDs/DVDs

Study Guides/Exam Preps/Board Reviews

Journals
■ Can be subscribed to as print copy or online or both
■ Trend is to electronic subscription only
■ Become familiar with the print collection; some publishers do not allow electronic access to journals until 6 to 12 months after publication
■ Ask about how to obtain articles not available at your institution

Journal Alerts
■ Services that scan the literature and send updates in a variety of electronic formats

- Designed to help clinicians stay up-to-date
- One popular example is Journal Watch, a free service from the publishers of the *New England Journal of Medicine*

Clinical Care Resources
- Provide clinically organized, evidence-based summaries for quick reference
- Examples include PIER (Physician Information and Education Resource), Dynamed, Up-To-Date, Essential Evidence Plus

The Medical Literature

The National Library of Medicine (NLM) is the producer of the world's premier biomedical database, MEDLINE. The subject scope of MEDLINE is biomedicine and health, including areas of the life sciences, behavioral sciences, chemical sciences, and bioengineering needed by health professionals and others engaged in basic research and clinical care, public health, health policy development, or related educational activities. MEDLINE contains 16 million references to articles, published from 1949 to the present, in more than 5000 current biomedical journals from the United States and over 80 foreign countries. A distinctive feature of MEDLINE is that the references are indexed with NLM's Medical Subject Headings (MeSH). MEDLINE can be searched for free using the NLM PubMed system. Although a growing number of MEDLINE references contain a link to the free full text of the article archived in an online repository called PubMed Central, or to other sites, you should take advantage of links to articles published in journals your library subscribes to by learning how to access PubMed through your library's Web page. Other vendors, such as MD Consult and OVID, offer access to the MEDLINE database, but the authors strongly recommend learning the PubMed interface because it is free and is provided by NLM, which is also the creator of the database. Using four of the five tabs on the PubMed search screen makes searching more efficient (Table 8-3).

TABLE 8-3

PubMed Search Tips

Limits	History	Clipboard	Details
■ Search by author and/or journal	■ Stores all your search statements for each search session	■ Allows you to combine search statements	■ Shows how the system translates your search into Medical Subject Headings (MeSH)
■ Limit retrieval by date, human or animal, language, publication types, ages of subjects, and more	■ Allows you to save references as you search	■ References saved in the Clipboard will be identified with a green number	■ Be sure to check the Details Tab for each concept you enter to learn MeSH headings and see that the system translated your search correctly
■ Do not limit to full-text, free full-text, or abstracts: you will miss relevant articles	■ The History will be cleared after a certain amount of inactivity (check with your library).	■ References can be printed or e-mailed in a variety of formats	■ To learn more about MESHs, click on the MeSH Browser from the blue sidebar on the left-hand side

Linking to Full-Text Articles from PubMed

MEDLINE is a database of references and abstracts, not full-text articles. A number of MEDLINE references contain a link to the free full-text of the article archived in an online repository called PubMed Central or to publisher's Web sites; for these references there will be an icon with a solid green or orange stripe at the top. It is important to learn how to link from PubMed to articles published in journals your library subscribes to by accessing PubMed through your library's Web page. Ask your librarian for assistance.

Free Resources

PubMed Central is the National Institutes of Health (NIH) free digital archive of biomedical and life sciences journal literature. The NIH Public Access Policy ensures that the public has access to published results of NIH funded research by requiring scientists to submit journal articles that arise from NIH funds to PubMed Central. There is a link to PubMed Central from the blue side bar in PubMed.

My NCBI is a free service available from the PubMed home page. Once you register it allows you to save searches and set up e-mail alerts for new content.

MedlinePlus is another free service offered by NLM. It provides consumer-oriented health information in English and Spanish that can be used for patient education. It is a good source for statistics, identifying relevant organizations and local resources.

The National Guidelines Clearinghouse is a large database of clinical practice guidelines sponsored by the Agency for Healthcare Research and Quality (AHRQ). It is searchable by topic or organization and has a feature that allows you to compare guidelines.

Clinical Trials.gov is a registry of federally and privately supported clinical trials conducted in the United States and around the world. It provides information about a trial's purpose, who may participate, locations, and phone numbers for more details. The registry is searchable by condition, drug intervention, sponsor, or locations. Information for patients about participating in clinical trials is also available.

Google is the most popular search engine, but Google Scholar is a better choice for searching the scholarly literature. Because it searches across many disciplines and sources, including theses, books, abstracts, and articles, it can be used in addition to PubMed. Some libraries provide a link to Google Scholar from their Web page.

Managing References

Reference management software allows you to download, store, track and cite reference information for presentations and publications. Products such as EndNote and Reference Manager are available, but many libraries purchase a site license for their institution. References in a bibliography always include author(s), article title, journal, volume, date and beginning page. Formats vary slightly between journals. One common standard is the Uniform Requirements for Manuscripts Submitted to Biomedical Journals from the International Committee of Medical Journal Editors.

Critically Evaluating the Medical Literature

Patrick C. Alguire

It is useful to understand the relative value of conclusions from different types of publications. The design of a study often limits the strength of the conclusions that can be drawn from it. Two of the most powerful study designs are systematic reviews and meta-analyses of the results of multiple randomized trials, such as those by the Cochrane Collaboration (http://www.cochrane.org). These reviews carefully combine data from multiple studies to draw conclusions that were impossible to determine from the individual, often smaller, studies.

Randomized controlled trials are also useful because they control for extraneous variables and, through blinding, for possible placebo effects. Applying evidence from a single randomized trial can be problematic because many of these early findings may not have been reproducible in subsequent studies. Multiple randomized trials that draw the same conclusion, or analyze multiple trials using meta-analysis techniques, provide more confidence in the findings.

Cohort studies (e.g., the Framingham study) follow many individuals for several years and typically control for extraneous variables. They are potentially useful but are more prone to bias because of how the subjects are recruited (nonrandom allocation).

Other study designs, such as case-control or case series, may be useful for generating hypotheses but have weaknesses inherent in their designs that hinder their ability to provide firm conclusions.

It is important to know whether the clinical information found during a literature search is evidence-based. Systematic review articles or meta-analyses that summarize the literature and describe the explicit article-selection criteria used are less likely to be biased in the selection of articles that support their conclusion than articles or meta-analyses that do not. These criteria should include a search of large bibliographic databases, such as MEDLINE and EMBASE (http://www.embase.com), and other measures to ensure that important studies have not been overlooked or improperly assessed.

Any source of information that provides specific clinical recommendations should also describe how the evidence was used to reach the stage of formal recommendation or guideline. Often, this process involves a system of letters and numbers representing each recommendation that reflects the amount and strength of the supporting evidence. For example, the U.S. Preventive Services Task Force (USPSTF; see http://www.ahrq.gov/) uses a system that reflects the strength for or against a given recommendation (A, B, C, D, I).

Although practice guidelines provide actual recommendations, the medical literature provides the data that inform the clinical decision-making process. Data are presented with measures of clinical significance. Beyond sensitivity, specificity, predictive value, and odds ratios, several newer epidemiologic measures are now used in research literature, meta-analyses, and review articles to describe the significance of diagnostic tests and the efficacy of treatments.

The utility of a diagnostic test has typically been represented by sensitivity and specificity. Sensitivity refers to the percentage of people with disease who are correctly diagnosed, whereas specificity refers to the percentage of people without disease who are correctly diagnosed. Based on sensitivity and specificity, the likelihood ratio (LR) has the advantage of summarizing in a single number the clinical utility of a test or physical examination finding. The LR is a function of a test, such as stress echocardiography, for confirming or excluding a diagnosis, such as coronary artery disease. The LR of a positive test or, a test that "rules in" a diagnosis, is calculated by the formula

$$\text{LR of positive test} = \text{sensitivity} / (1 - \text{specificity})$$

whereas the LR of a negative test, or a test that "rules out" a diagnosis, is calculated by the formula

$$\text{LR of negative test} = (1 - \text{sensitivity}) / \text{specificity}$$

The pretest probability refers to the percentage of patients who have the target disorder as determined before the test is performed. The farther away the LR is from 1.0, the more clinically useful a test is in increasing or decreasing the pretest probability for confirming or excluding the target disorder. An LR between 1 and 3 for a positive test indicates a less useful test than one with an LR between 5 and 7. For example, a positive result for a test with an LR of 8 adds approximately 40% to the pretest probability that a patient has a specific diagnosis. Positive LRs of 2, 5, and 10 increase the probability of disease by 15%, 30%, and 45%, respectively. Negative LRs of 0.5, 0.2, and 0.1 decrease the probability of disease by 15%, 30%, and 45%, respectively. When the pretest probability is very low or very high, only an extremely high LR would be needed to influence management decisions. Diagnostic tests are most useful when the pretest probability is within the intermediate range.

The number needed to treat (NNT), which represents the effect of treatments on patients, indicates how many patients must receive a treatment to produce one additional improved outcome compared with the control treatment. The NNT is calculated from the absolute risk reduction (ARR), which is the difference in outcome observed between the placebo and active treatment. This is different from the relative risk reduction (RRR), which is a ratio of the difference in outcome between placebo and active treatment. The NNT is calculated by taking the inverse of the ARR, or the difference between event rates of patients who received treatment and those who did not. For example, if myocardial infarction occurred in 10% of patients in a clinical trial who received an experimental medication designed to prevent myocardial infarction, compared with 20% of patients who received placebo, the RRR would be 0.5 (0.1/0.2), the ARR would be 0.10 (0.2 − 0.1), and the NNT would be 10, the inverse of 0.20 − 0.10 (or, 1/0.1). This means that 10 patients would need to be treated to prevent one myocardial infarction with the use of the new medication. The lower the NNT, the more effective is the treatment.

Most studies now provide estimates of event rates in terms of confidence intervals (CI). This number, which is a real calculation of events that occurred in a study, indicates that if a study were repeated 100 times, a result within the specified range of values would be expected 95% of the time (when using a 95% CI). In studies, this is typically represented by a number, followed by a parenthetical range of two other numbers, for example, "4.5 (95% CI, 3.8 to 5.4)". Therefore, if a study's result were 4.5, and the study were repeated 100 times, 95% of the time the result would be between 3.8 and 5.4. Larger studies typically have narrower CIs.

Research Sponsored by Pharmaceutical Companies

In the United States, the pharmaceutical industry is a billion-dollar business. Pharmaceutical firms are anxious to develop and bring to market new drugs which in addition to meeting real needs to provide and improve patient care, may bring hefty profits to the companies that develop them. New drug development requires a great deal of research, and American pharmaceutical companies invest very heavily in this research.

When reviewing medical literature or evaluating drug information from any source, it is important to identify if and to what degree the research is being supported by a pharmaceutical company that is anxious to develop or encourage the use of the drug. Authors are required to disclose any such affiliations. Pharmaceutically sponsored research certainly can be and most often is valid and ethical, and a great deal of the credit for advances in medicine should rightly be given to those firms. At the same time, there is always a potential conflict of interest when the sponsor of the research has the potential to profit by the approval and/or use of the drug which it manufactures. For that reason, drug trials and other research sponsored by pharmaceutical firms should be scrutinized most carefully and corroborating data and research from other sources should be sought before the conclusions proffered by the authors of pharmaceutically sponsored research are accepted.

Simulation in Medical Education

Antoinette Spevetz

> I hear, I forget;
> I see, I remember;
> I do, I understand.
> —*Chinese proverb*

Of the many challenges in medical education today perhaps the most difficult is allowing trainees the opportunity to learn patient care skills while actively providing patient care. When a trainee becomes anxious and appears uncomfortable and unsure of himself or herself, the patient may sense that the trainee is new to medicine or the procedure and become anxious as well. It is difficult for the experienced clinician to address the trainee in front of the patient, pointing out both what was done well and what was not done well. There is no opportunity for practice and reflection on the situation at hand. This is particularly difficult when teaching procedural skills and even more so with the awake patient.

This issue was moved to the forefront in 1999 with the release of the landmark report on medical errors and patient safety by the United States Institute of Medicine entitled "To Error is Human: Building a Safer Health System." The report implies that medical errors are a leading cause of death in the United States and total preventable costs were estimated between 17 and 29 billion dollars. This report recommended the development of patient safety initiatives and has helped to drive the use of simulation in medical education.

Simulation was first used in 1922 by Edward Link for use in flight simulation. In 1960-1970 it became the standard in training in commercial aviation, nuclear power production, in military interventions and by National Aeronautics and Space Administration (NASA). In the airline industry, a 99.99% reliability rate would be unacceptable, predicting an accident every 20 days at large regional airports. With the use of simulation, pilots can repeatedly practice rare crisis scenarios, so, should an actual crisis occur, their responses would be automatic. Crew resource management (CRM) is a formal program that concentrates on the human factors in aviation. While pilots were technically competent, their people skills were deficient. CRM allows the pilot to improve communication, prioritize tasks, delegate authority, and monitor automated equipment.

In medicine, anesthesia has been a leader in the use of simulation. Dangers associated with anesthesia were brought to the forefront by a television documentary entitled "Deep Sleep" where morbidity and mortality was estimated at a rate of 1.7:10,000 cases.

It was found that two thirds of anesthesia incidents were secondary to human performance errors and of these 82% were preventable. Parallels were seen between the aviation industry and the practice of anesthesia. Since this time the use of simulation has expanded to use in all facets of medicine, surgery, nursing, and paramedical education.

Simulation is a technique to replace or amplify real experiences with guided experiences that evoke or replicate substantial aspects of the real world in a fully interactive and immersive manner. The advantages of simulation are many. In simulation the patients are neither harmed or at risk for harm. There are no real-time constraints other than those of the learner and teacher. It allows the opportunity to start and stop the session with real-time feedback. It also gives the learner an opportunity to commit an error with no immediate feedback, allowing him or her to see what happens when incorrect choices are made. Relatively rare occurrences can be practiced over and over in this simulated setting. This method allows for team training as well as individual training. It is useful for both novices and experts because complexity can be controlled and learners can reflect on their performance and receive feedback.

Laerdal developed the original Resusci Anne model years ago in collaboration with Peter Safar and Bjorn Lind with the intention of facilitating resuscitation skills by using a life-like model. This basic model continues to be used in Advanced and Basic Life Support courses all over the world.

The range of simulation resources now available includes

- Simple task trainers that usually have few moving parts and provide little feedback
- Standardized patients (SPs) that role play scenarios and can give feedback on communication skills and physical examination technique
- Computer-based programs using virtual reality with high-fidelity audio-visual effects
- High-fidelity patient care models

The last provides an anatomically correct, fully programmable adult or pediatric training platform capable of responding to therapeutic intervention. When linked to a computer, full-body manikins like SimMan (Laerdal), the Human Patient Simulator (HPS, METI) and others may be controlled automatically or manually by the facilitator, and instructors can even role play the patient by speaking through the manikin. One can palpate a pulse, listen to breath sounds, heart tones, place a central line, defibrillate, and attempt to intubate a difficult airway. The manikin can then be restored to a healthy patient again and again to practice training skills over and over.

Simulation is used to teach airway management including bay valve mask techniques and intubation. Some of the mannequins are able to mimic a swollen airway, trismus, and closed vocal cords. Another practical use of simulation is for practice of procedural skills such as central line placement, chest tube placement, and decompression of the pneumothorax. Their design allows repeated practice of the procedure until the students are comfortable and competent.

In the simulation exercise, the students are provided an introduction to the process and to the manikin. A clinical scenario is given to them and they are expected to perform as they would in the actual clinical situation. They are able to take a history, examine the "patient," and monitor changing vital signs that respond to the treatment given. The scenarios are recorded on video, allowing the student to review his or her performance.

When the scenario is complete the participants are debriefed, allowing them to comment on their performance, view the tape and learn from their mistakes. Communication techniques are emphasized to prevent error. Directions should be given to a specific person, and the receiver should repeat back what has been heard. These techniques have been found beneficial in other industries as well.

The simulation exercise also allows practice of team-building skills. While one may know the steps of advanced cardiac life support (ACLS), they often have no experience with managing a team of people. Effective teams are a key to achieving high performance.

Patients clearly benefit from the use of simulation in that adverse events are reduced and outcomes are improved. We have the technology, the ability, and the responsibility to provide our patients with the highest quality care available. The use of simulation in these high-risk, low-frequency events is invaluable to both the patient and the practitioner. As simulation technology advances and become integrated into all facets of medical education, there will come a day when the phrase "I've never done that" will no longer be spoken. Students and residents will have had the opportunity to practice patient scenarios, crisis intervention, and procedures long before caring for their first patient.

PROFESSIONALISM AND ETHICAL ISSUES

Christy A. Rentmeester

Confidentiality

Western medicine in American society tends to try to maintain sharp distinctions between public and private dimensions of life. This has important implications regarding patients' health information. Generally, information pertaining to patients' health is private and, therefore, protected; this means that all health care professionals are expected to keep patients' health information confidential. Patients expect that they can trust physicians to keep their health information confidential, and patients' willingness to reveal clinically relevant details about their lives often depend upon whether they trust their physicians.

What can physicians do to honor the confidentiality of a patient's health information? Generally, physicians must obtain patient permission to discuss any aspects of his or her care with others. Physicians are also expected to restrict discussion about patient care to their professional environment and to avoid discussing their patients in public places (cafeterias and elevators, for example). When physicians are asked questions about their patients by others (family, friends, and members of the media, for example), they are expected to obtain patient consent before disclosing any details of condition or care.

However, even conscientious physicians astutely aware of the importance of confidentiality in their relationships with patients, face interesting, important, and complex questions about whether and when to keep patients' protected health information confidential. Cases in which it might be justifiable for physicians to disclose information about a patient are those involving public health risks from communicable diseases. For example, physicians are generally not required to "report" patients with HIV. (HIV status is protected health information, and patients would be unlikely to trust physicians with intimate information about IV drug use or sexual practices if they suspected their physicians would disclose their HIV status.) But physicians can have what are called duties to warn other people (sexual partners, for example) if they think those people might be at risk of harm by their patient. In these cases, caregivers who can identify specific individuals that have been exposed to HIV or are at risk for being exposed to HIV by their patient can get help carrying out this duty to warn those at risk. Some states, for example, support processes by which physicians can ask for the assistance of the State Department of Health or the State Epidemiologist in informing specific individuals suspected to be at risk for contracting HIV and in encouraging those individuals to seek HIV testing and support services.

Informed Consent

A patient's informed consent to a treatment or procedure is what authorizes a physician to initiate or perform that treatment or procedure. There are legal consequences to failing to obtain informed consent, and such failure can generate distrust of physicians by patients. Consent is often documented with a patient's written signature, but patients often consent verbally, too. In either case, informed consent should be a shared process of information exchange between a patient and health care professional that expresses respect for patient autonomy and support for patients making difficult and sometimes life-altering decisions. For consent to, or refusal of, a procedure or treatment to be valid, the patient must

1. Understand the risks and benefits of that procedure or treatment
2. Understand the consequences of consenting to or foregoing that procedure or treatment
3. Understand alternatives to a particular procedure or treatment
4. Consent or refuse voluntarily

Physicians should encourage patients to ask questions about risks, benefits, and goals of treatment, give them time to think carefully about their options, and ask patients about their concerns, fears, and moral values. When presenting information to patients, physicians should avoid use of medical jargon and acronyms, solicit the assistance of interpreters when necessary, and clarify their recommendations.

Sometimes, whether a patient's consent is voluntary depends upon whether that patient has decision-making capacity. Patients have decision-making capacity when they can understand information, express preferences, and make choices consistent with values they've expressed in the past. If a patient lacks decision-making capacity for a particular decision, physicians should identify an appropriate surrogate (or proxy) decision-maker (sometimes a patient's loved one or friend, for example). However, even if patients do not have the capacity to make serious decisions about risky procedures and treatments, they may have the capacity to make other decisions about procedures and treatments with less risk. In other words, a patient's decision-making capacity is evaluated for a particular decision at one particular point in time.

Patients suspected of having compromised decision-making capacity must be carefully assessed. It is noteworthy that physicians are far more likely to question patients' decision-making capacity when patients refuse treatments that physicians recommend, particularly if those treatments prolong biological life (see the references by Masand et al and Luce). Whether procedures and treatments in end-of-life care prolong patients' lives or prolong their deaths is a matter of ethical and clinical debate, but when a patient's decision-making capacity is questioned because patients' preferences conflict with physicians' advice, important questions surface about imbalances of power between physicians and patients and the conditions under which patients have their preferences taken seriously.

Surrogate decision-makers typically try to make decisions in the best interests of patients and generally try to make decisions that express the patient's values. In some cases, however, surrogate decision-makers and caregivers disagree about the terms in which a patient's best interests and patient's values should be defined. In these cases, physicians can request consultation from the hospital or clinic's Ethics Consultation Service or try to facilitate discussion and understanding among patients' loved ones and caregivers about what's clinically and ethically at stake for that particular patient, clarify the goals of procedures and treatments for that particular patient, and consider whether and when the procedures and treatments promote goals that are consistent with values, as defined by the patient.

Respect, Autonomy, and Self-Determination

In health care, respecting patients and their autonomy means honoring their rights to self-determination. A common misconception is that respect for patient autonomy simply means giving patients what they want. This is misguided, however, because patients and physicians do not have equal knowledge about the conditions that affect a patient's health. For example, a patient who has a virus and demands antibiotics will not be helped by a physician who just gives that patient what he or she wants; antibiotics do not cure viral infections. Respecting patient autonomy begins with listening carefully to patients without interrupting them and asking them to express their health care goals.

Another way for a physician to express respect for patient autonomy and rights to self-determination is to take patient claims about what they know about their illnesses, experiences, and bodies seriously. Perhaps you wonder, "Why wouldn't a physician take patients' claims seriously?" But, when patient symptoms do not fit well into medical models of thinking about illness and disease, some physicians question whether patients know what they are talking about. Idiopathic diagnoses—those made when the diagnoses physicians have been trained to identify and understand have been eliminated—often expose the limitations of medical models of thinking about patient suffering. Chronic fatigue syndrome (CFS), for example, is an idiopathic diagnosis, and patients with CFS are sometimes accused of making up experiences of fatigue. When physicians discount patients' legitimate claims about what they know about their illness or what they experience, they undermine patient autonomy.

There are important exceptions to the general rule that patients have rights to self-determination regarding their health care decisions. Patients with compromised decision-making capacity, for example, are especially vulnerable and require physicians to consider whether and when they ought to be considered autonomous. On the other hand, there are classes of patients whose autonomy is sometimes unjustifiably questioned by physicians. Patients with mental illnesses, for example, are often assumed to have less decision-making authority. While this might be acceptable in some cases for patients with severe mental illnesses, it does not follow that there is good reason to question the autonomy of all chronically mentally ill patients or patients with moderate or mild mental illnesses. Patients with severe acute pain or chronic pain conditions who need narcotics to properly control their pain are another group of patients whose autonomy is sometimes unjustifiably undermined. This is because they are frequently suspected of being drug addicts who are not in "real" pain. It is difficult to reliably discern differences between patients who are in pain and patients who seek narcotics because they are addicts. Furthermore, patients who are addicts still suffer pain and deserve to have their pain treated. This remains a persistent conceptual and practical problem in clinical medical practice.

Elderly patients, children, and patients with disabilities are other groups of patients who can unjustifiably be perceived by physicians as having less autonomy. Additionally, patients perceived as members of racial and ethnic minority groups or patients who have spiritual beliefs that are uncommon in "mainstream" American culture are also sometimes inappropriately seen as being less authoritative and capable decision-makers. Patients with poor English language skills, who are unable to articulate their preferences clearly, may also be perceived as having less autonomy, perhaps because physicians have to work harder to understand them.

Autonomy is rooted in traditions of American individualism and might be a less prominent issue for patients whose cultural background is more communitarian than individualistic. In these cases, physicians' relationships with patients and their loved ones are of utmost importance.

LEARNING WITHIN THE TEAM SYSTEM

Vijay Rajput and Christy A. Rentmeester

We now turn to discussion of teams and the roles residents play on teams within the system of patient care and graduate medical education in the United States. We use the word "team" regularly in conversation about health care. For example, there are code teams, surgical teams, and consultation teams. Teams are groups of people who work toward a common goal within organizations. Team members are interdependent, share responsibility for tasks and outcomes, and manage relationships across organizational and departmental boundaries (Cohen and Bailey 1997). In health care, a team is a group of professional caregivers, each of whom is trained to use different methods and tools to care for patients, who organize and divide the labor of caring for patients. Continuous clear communication among team members and frequent reflection on how team members work together are critical for teams to operative effectively and efficiently. Teams need to express emotional intelligence and act compassionately toward patients. The following are key features of a team whose members work well together: team identity, motivation, emotional awareness, communication, stress tolerance, ability to resolve conflicts, and the ability to sustain a positive mood (Hughes and Terrell 2007).

Multidisciplinary teams of professionals have been critical in the United States for about 50 years. During this time, standards for how to care for patients have evolved, and these standards are taught to residents by team leaders, who earn their positions of leadership through experience. As you gain experience, you gain more rank and authority on the team. Rank is not the only important element of team membership, however. Multidisciplinarity is a key feature of the learning environments for health care trainees, and different types of team members other than physicians (nurses, therapists, and pharmacists, for example) and their roles are described in other chapters. As residents, one part of your role will be to collaborate to discuss plans for how to care for patients.

In 2001, the Institute of Medicine's Committee on the Quality of Health Care in America released its report *Crossing the Quality Chasm: A New Health System for the 21st Century*, which called for improvement in our health care system. The report stated that while team practice is common, the training of health care professionals is still typically compartmentalized by discipline. Other significant challenges one needs to be aware of to be an effective team member and resident in the American health care system are listed in Box 8-7.

☑ **BOX 8-7   Challenges for IMGs in Adapting to Residency Training and American Health Care**

- Historically subordinate roles of women to men in American society
- Historically subordinate roles of nurses to physicians in American health care
- States' authority to regulate physician licensure
- Differences in type and quality of residents' medical educations
- Differences in residents' styles of learning
- Differences in patterns of personal and professional socialization
- Differences in residents' language and communication skills
- Need to adapt to new cultural, social, and professional environments

---

Crossing the Quality Chasm notes that failure to address these challenges and to work well as a team can lead to failures in the continuity of patient care and can limit physician opportunities to see their patients holistically. For example, historically women's social roles have been subordinate to men's roles in American society, and nurses have been subordinate to physicians in American health care. Residents can easily make all colleagues, regardless of gender or professional roles, feel that their professional knowledge and expertise are important and critical to delivering good care to patients by inviting diverse opinions and perspectives into processes of decision-making. Contrary to television portrayals of physicians, physicians are not "captains" or "quarterbacks" of the health care team. Rather, skilled physicians express leadership on the health care team by acknowledging that everyone should work together for the best possible patient care and by depending upon the knowledge, skill, and expertise of colleagues in, for example, nursing and pharmacy.

Differences in the type and quality of resident medical education can also be a challenge. IMG degrees come from different medical schools from all over the world. It is not necessarily the case that one is better than the other, but the nature and scope of knowledge and expertise imparted by each of these programs can vary dramatically. Also, there is no single way to learn medicine, and residents will have many different styles of learning new material, as well as different styles of adapting to new cultural, social, and professional environments. Another common challenge for IMGs is that individual states in the United States license physicians. Sometimes the licensure process is time consuming and cumbersome. Begin your process of applying for appropriate licensure early and work with your residency program director to facilitate this process.

The Accreditation Council for Graduate Medical Education (ACGME) Outcome Project calls upon all residency programs to require residents to develop competencies in six specific areas. Some of its objectives refer to expectations of resident physicians:

> [R]esidents are expected ... to work with health care professionals, including those from other disciplines, to provide patient-focused care ... to work effectively with others as a member or leader of a health care team ... to understand how their patient care and other professional practices affect other health care professionals ... and to know how to partner with health care managers and health care providers to assess, coordinate, and improve health care.

The Graduate Medical Education Core Curriculum of the Association of American Medical Colleges (AAMC) has goals for training residents that include cultivating their "abilit[ies] to work in team settings by defining roles and tasks, planning and prioritizing, accepting responsibilities, and helping others" (AAMC Core Curriculum Working Group 2000). Residents are also expected to "demonstrate skills of conflict resolution," including listening and explaining, offering feedback, expressing respect, earning trust, and cultivating consensus among team members. Physicians that support and build effective teams can improve the quality of care patients receive and enhance patient safety. Although it might not be obvious to IMGs new to the American team approach to health care, patients and their loved ones are essential team members. Physicians must skillfully draw upon the experiences of patients and their loved ones as they offer and exchange information and develop care plans. Patients and their loved ones play important roles in health care decision-making and care management.

Teamwork can reduce individual workloads, reduce burnout among house staff members, and help individuals comply with standards about work hours. Teams work effectively when they have clear purposes, good communication, are well coordinated, and develop processes for resolving disagreements. Active participation of all team members is essential for successful outcomes for patient care and learning. Team trust and interdependence are also benefits of working together; they produce and are produced by accountability of the group.

Graduated Levels of Responsibilities for Patient Care and Teaching

Your role as intern or resident is to supervise patient care, set goals for the teams, and coordinate care with other teams and health care professionals. As an IMG, you might not have a lot of experience with team dynamics. Generally, a health care team comprises a variety of learners with different degrees of experience. You will be given more responsibilities for managing patient care as your level of experience increases. After you have earned your doctorate degree in medicine, your first role on the health care team is as an intern, a first-year resident, also called a post-graduate year 1 (PGY1) resident.

As an intern, you start lowest in hierarchy of all physicians on health care teams. Mainly, your team will rely on you to provide reports and updates about patients. More experienced residents, chief residents, and attending physicians are your teachers and supervisors. One of your important roles is to help your team identify and avoid errors. You are the key team member who communicates in conferences with other health care professionals, such as nurses, social workers, physical therapists, and pharmacists. As you gain more experience, you might represent your department in conferences or grand rounds. Additionally, your communication skills and professionalism count importantly towards overall patient satisfaction scores that hospitals report to the public. Throughout your training, you will be given reports on quality, patient safety, and other goals and initiatives within the organization where you work (Table 8-4).

Teaching Responsibilities

As new team members, you also communicate with attending physicians and teach students and other learners who are less experienced than you. Learning of clinical skill and clinical comportment occurs at patients' bedsides and from peers. Typically, programs emphasize the establishment of proactive, systematic approaches to developing and improving team-based performance through direct observation and timely feedback to

TABLE 8-4

Features of an Effective Health Care Team

Features	Comments
Clear goals and roles	As an intern or resident working in the hospital, you should have clear goals about care for each patient and a clear understanding of your own responsibilities in learning and teaching. As a team, identify goals of care for patients, goals for learning as team, and set clear expectations for each other (e.g., senior residents should ask each intern and student about what needs to be done before morning report).
Collegiality	Effective, efficient work flow and outcomes are optimal when everyone on the team cultivates collegial relationships with each other.
Active participation	All members of your team should participate actively in effective patient care, learning, and teaching. Your active participation is critical when your role is to provide leadership to students and other junior team members.
Attentive listening	Attentive listening to all team members and taking their views about patient care seriously are essential. In the United States, nurses and other health care professionals play key roles in actively managing patient care.
Respectful expression of disagreement	When you do not agree with a colleague's opinion, you must find a civil, professional way to express disagreement. Good patient care is a goal you share in common with your fellow professionals; try to draw upon this to resolve disagreement. Attending, resident, and consultant physicians, for example, will not always agree on how best to manage a patient's care. Reasonable physicians can disagree, and skilled physicians find ways to openly, collegially discuss important differences of opinion, keeping the best interests of patients in mind.
Maintain open communication about errors and unanticipated poor outcomes	Open communication calls for transparency among team members, patients, and their loved ones. As described in other chapters, open communication among all team members is essential to achieve the best outcomes for patients. Particularly in cases in which outcomes are poor or errors have occurred, however, open disclosure of information is important to patients and their loved ones. Disclosure of errors and unanticipated poor outcomes is usually done as a team, and as an intern or resident you should always inform your senior resident and attending physician when they occur.
Shared leadership and mentoring	As an intern, you will be assigned an important role in managing information about patient care and you will also teach, support, and offer feedback to medical students and other junior team members. You should try, whenever possible, to acknowledge the effort and work of other team members and draw upon their capabilities and strengths.
Manage relationships among fellow professionals in the hospital system	You will commonly have to work with teams other than your own while managing patient care in the hospital. As a member of a night float team, for example, you will work closely with an Emergency Department team to admit patients. You will also manage communication with nurses, pharmacists, therapists, and social workers, and you will need to adapt as teams routinely change membership.
Cultural competence	U.S. health care teams are typically socially and culturally diverse groups of people. Like you, some team members will have received their medical educations outside the United States. Like you, they will bring different styles to working with a team or independently. Learn to understand these differences.
Self-awareness	Cultivating awareness about how you express your emotions and your styles of using body language when communicating can help you avoid misunderstanding and conflict as you work with your team.

trainees. Recently, the ACGME held its first conference on designing effective health care learning environments; one common theme was teaching residents to be helpful and reliable team members.

Teaching Medical and Other Health Professions Students

In the United States, medical students are active learners at the bedside. William Osler (1849-1919) incorporated the art of patient care with the science of diagnosis and medical teaching. He introduced different levels of education, including live-in resident staff with different degrees of experience in caring for patients. This gave rise to clerkships in early 20th century. Medical students spend their third and fourth years of medical school in clerkships in which they rotate through different medical specialties. Medical students will need your guidance in taking histories, learning how to physically examine patients, and learning how to write progress notes in patients' charts, for example. Medical students round as team members on the floors with residents of all levels.

Teaching Junior Residents

As residents advance in experience, their attending physicians give them more sophisticated responsibilities. Senior residents mentor junior residents and medical students and gain more experience teaching, too. Senior residents are also expected to give more formal presentations to their colleagues as they progress in their training.

Another important thing residents learn throughout their training is when to acknowledge limitations in their own knowledge and skill and how and when to draw upon the expertise of their colleagues to help patients. For example, physicians frequently request consultations from colleagues who are known for their expertise and experience in specific areas of clinical practice. Consultations are opportunities to learn about how to care better for a patient from an expert, whom you request to advise you and your team.

Although physicians do not always agree with one another or with the advice of experts, these disagreements are also opportunities for learning. Physicians need to cultivate skills in collegially exchanging views about the reasons certain treatments or procedures should or should not be offered to a patient. "One of the goals of reason exchange is to try to forge consensus about the reasons for acting in a clinical situation" (Rentmeester 2007). Forging consensus and agreement about how to help patients requires that physicians are well trained in how to collegially negotiate differences in their views of what constitutes appropriate care for patients.

Self-Study

Vijay Rajput and Christy A. Rentmeester

Residents in internal medicine programs, for example, typically have about 150 hours of didactic (lecture and classroom-based) learning sessions; these include morning report, noon conferences, and grand rounds. Of course, a lot of learning also occurs while rounding at patients' bedsides. Additionally, all trainees (medical students, interns, and residents) need to cultivate skills in finding pertinent, recent medical literature to help their teams decide what kind of care to offer patients. In addition to preparing for state licensure and specialty board examinations, you need to develop the skills of a self-motivated, lifelong learner because standards of care and evidence-based justifications for standards of care will continually evolve throughout your career as a physician.

Residency programs typically provide in-service training sessions about specialty board examinations for their residents each year. Adequate preparation for specialty board examinations also requires study of standard textbooks, reviews in journals, and materials prepared by your specialty society specifically for these high-stakes examinations. Commercial board preparation materials are also available. Because it is impossible to read all current journal articles in your field, an excellent alternative strategy is reading about specific clinical problems and questions raised in the course of caring for your patients. Some residents commonly carry index cards or personal digital assistants (PDAs) to help them store and manage clinically relevant information. Residents also commonly draw upon Web-based resources, like PubMed, Google, ACP Journal Club, BMJ Updates, InfoPOEMS, Up-To-Date and other databases for literature searches and catalogues of clinical facts.

Remember, however, more information does not mean more knowledge. You still need to make decisions about, and assess what constitutes, important and reliable information. That is, in many cases, it's less important for you to memorize information than it is for you to have solid, rigorous skills in identifying pertinent questions, identifying ways to probe those questions productively, and accessing information in a timely fashion. Librarians can be tremendously helpful; ask them for help with particular queries and draw upon their expertise and training in information management. Most importantly, develop a strategy for reserving self-study time for yourself throughout your residency.

Research Opportunities Before and During Residency

Vani Dandolu

BEFORE RESIDENCY: HOW DOES RESEARCH HELP IMGS?

Research experience is one criterion (along with examination scores, year of graduation, recommendation letters, and Dean's letter) used by program directors to select residents. A published manuscript or abstract presented at a national or regional meeting is good documentation of research participation. Be prepared to explain your role in the research proposal, which may include activities such as reviewing the literature; developing the research design and study plan; obtaining IRB (institutional review board) approval; data collection, entry, and analysis; and writing the manuscript. Having another degree (e.g., MPH) or experience with the use of statistical software (e.g., SAS, SPSS, Stata) is an additional desired asset.

Research outside of the United States is not given much credit unless it results in presentation at a scientific meeting or peer-reviewed publication or poster presentation. Most-peer reviewed journals are cited in the National Library of Medicine's PubMed. You can also check the scholarly value of the journal by its impact factor, which can be obtained using Journal Citation Reports (JCR), a database available through most libraries. The impact factor is a calculation of how many times a particular article has been cited in other articles.

HOW DO I GET INVOLVED IN A RESEARCH PROJECT?

There are several ways of finding research mentors. The most direct is to explore the Web sites of residency programs for listings of faculty and their research area of interest; often this information will also include the faculty's publications. You may also make appointments with faculty to discuss your interest in his/her area of work. Some faculty may have research funding available, but if you entered the United States on a student visa or an employment-based visa and are not eligible for funding, you can participate as a volunteer. Depending upon your level of involvement, you may be eligible for co-authorship and at the very least a letter of recommendation at the end of your participation.

If you are not confined to any specific geographic area and you have a Green Card or visa to work in the United States, you can explore opportunities at the major academic health care institutions to find funded investigators in the field of your interest. Many of them are well-versed with the process of mentoring residents and students and have rigorous research training in their field of interest.

You may wish to consider beginning your medical career in the United States as a research fellow. These are paid research training opportunities that can be obtained from abroad. However, if you get J-1 visa sponsored for a research fellowship, it may be difficult to change your status for residency training. Nevertheless, experience as a research fellow may facilitate your entry into highly competitive clinical fellowships, particularly if the research fellowship is affiliated with the clinical fellowship training program.

NIH, HRSA, and Private Industry

Federal funding from the National Institutes of Health and Health Resources and Services Administration offers research and training opportunities in a wide variety of medicine disciplines. These are primarily institutional grants and enable institutions to provide a stipend and a training allowance to the faculty. These grants, however, are only available for U.S. citizens and permanent residents.

The Pharmaceutical Research and Manufacturers of America (PhRMA) represents the country's leading pharmaceutical research and biotechnology companies and is a major source of funding for research related to drugs.

Academic Integrity and Scientific Integrity

The practice of medicine and science requires honesty, objectivity, and collegiality. In 1993, the NIH revitalization act established the Commission on Research Integrity to address scientific misconduct.

Plagiarism is the use of another person's labor, ideas, or words without acknowledging the source. If a body of work has entailed consulting other resources (e.g., journals, books, other media), these resources must be cited, including the organization of ideas, ideas themselves, or actual language. Failure to acknowledge the source of borrowed material is plagiarism. Undocumented use of materials from the World Wide Web is plagiarism. Plagiarism is the most common type of academic misconduct of health professionals. In response to these growing problems, many schools and colleges have honor codes and associated policy and guidelines relating to scientific and academic integrity and honesty. The concerns about scientific and academic misconduct extend beyond the laboratory and clinic and have immediate relevance for the IMG. Personal statements submitted for application must represent original and truthful facts about your private and professional life. Misrepresentation of your private and professional life is unprofessional behavior that can exclude you from training in the United States.

Many IMGs are not aware of the regulations involving scientific writing. If this is the case for you, it may be worth your time to take any one of many online courses on academic integrity and plagiarism before embarking on a research project. Additionally, every major institution conducting biomedical research provides self-learning modules or access to other educational resources such as the one by National Cancer Institute. You may wish to explore http://www.plagiarism.org to learn more about plagiarism. Other plagiarism-detection software and services can be found at http://www.tunitin.com.

Research Misconduct

Research misconduct is significant misbehavior related to improper use of intellectual property, failing to acknowledge contributors, intentionally impeding research endeavors, or false documentation or presentation of research in oral or written formats.

The Office of Research Integrity (ORI) Web site has information and educational materials, such as the ORI Introduction to the Responsible Conduct of Research. The Responsible Conduct of Research Education Consortium hosts an excellent Web site with many resources for administrators and teachers, including well-developed case studies.

ORI supports several programs designed to promote education and training in the responsible conduct of research that covers the following nine instructional areas:

- Data acquisition, management, sharing and ownership
- Conflict of interest and commitment
- Human subjects
- Animal welfare
- Research misconduct
- Publication practices and responsible authorship
- Mentor/trainee responsibilities
- Peer review
- Collaborative science

More information on these programs can be obtained directly from the ORI Web site at http://ori.dhhs.gov/education.

The Council of Graduate Schools also has launched a major initiative to enhance the training of graduate students in the responsible conduct of research. The CGS initiative stems from a growing concern that many, if not most, students, postdoctoral fellows, technicians, and even faculty, arrive in the laboratory not fully informed about the norms of science, the ethical requirements of research, or the policies and regulations that govern research in the United States. More information on these issues can be obtained at http://www.cgsnet.org.

Participation in Research During Residency

Demonstration of resident participation in research is an important criterion for documentation of scholarly activity of residents in ACGME-accredited training programs. The ultimate goal of most residency-based research programs is to introduce residents to a process of organized inquiry and research. Residents may benefit by learning critical reading skills, participating in thoughtful inquiry, and learning about the rudiments of study design, project planning, and statistics. In some of these programs, residents plan and execute their own projects, with the advice and supervision of faculty mentors.

In training programs with a research requirement or opportunity, protected time is provided during the residency to work on a research project. Many programs will provide workshops or personal mentoring that introduces the resident to the rudiments of scientific inquiry, study design, planning, data collection, analysis, and oral and written presentation skills. Residents may have an opportunity to document their scholarly activities at national and regional meetings by presenting posters or papers; some may even lead to publication in peer-reviewed journals. This is excellent training for a career in medicine, because it gives you first-hand knowledge of how research is done and important insights on how to critically read original research articles. Finally, participation in research during the residency program is one way to improve your chances entering a highly competitive fellowship program.

References

Web Sites

Health Care Access for Uninsured Adults. Holahan and Spillman. The Urban Institute; Jan. 2002. Go to http://www.ahrq.gov/news/ulp/buyright/indicattr.htm.

http://www.acgme.org/acWebsite/home/home.asp.

http://www.healthaffairs.org.

http://cms.hhs.gov.

http://www.nj.gov/health.

http://www.va.gov.

Books and Journals

Accreditation Council for Graduate Medical Education. ACGME Outcome Project; 2007. Web site: http://www.acgme.org/outcome/.

Association of American Medical Colleges, Core Curriculum Working Group. Graduate Medical Education Core Curriculum. Washington, DC: AAMC; 2000.

Cohen SG, Bailey DR. What makes teams work: group effectiveness research from the shop floor to the executive suite. J Management. 1997;23:238-90.

Committee on Quality of Health Care in America. Crossing the Quality Chasm: A New Health System for the 21st Century. Institute of Medicine; 2001.

Cone DC, Alexander V, Myint W. EMTALA knowledge among on-call specialists at an academic medical center. J Emerg Med. 2006;30:444-6.

DeVita MA, Schaefer J, Lutz J, et al. Improving medical crisis team performance. Crit Care Med. 2004;32(2 Suppl):S61-5.

Grenvik A, Schaefer J. From Resusci-Anne to Sim-Man: the evolution of simulators in medicine. Crit Care Med. 2004;32(2 Suppl):S56-7.

Henley E. Medicare update: what the latest changes will mean for you. J Fam Pract. 2007;56:E1-3.

Hughes M, Terrell JB. The Emotionally Intelligent Team. New York: Wiley; 2007.

Iglehart JK. The American health care system: Medicare. N Engl J Med. 1999;340:327-32.

Iglehart JK. The dilemma of Medicaid. N Engl J Med. 2003;348:2140-8.

Kohn LT, Corrigan JM, Donaldson MS, eds. To Error is Human: Building a Safer Health System. Washington, DC: Institute of Medicine, National Academy Press; 1999.

Luce JM. Three patients who asked that life support be withheld or withdrawn in the surgical intensive care unit. Crit Care Med. 2002;30:775-80.

Masand PS, Bouckoms AJ, Fischel SV, et al. A prospective multicenter study of competency evaluations by psychiatric consultation services. Psychosomatics. 1998;39:55-60.

Owens JA, Avidan A, Baldwin D, Landrigan C. Improving sleep hygiene. Arch Intern Med. 2007;167:1738-44.

Philibert I, ed. Simulation and Rehearsal. ACGM Bulletin No. 2205; Dec. 2005.

Philibert I, Friedmann P, Williams WT, ACGME Work Group on Resident Duty Hours. New requirements for resident duty hours. JAMA. 2002;288:1112-4.

Rentmeester CA. "Why aren't you doing what we want?" Cultivating collegiality and communication between specialist and generalist physicians and residents. J Medical Ethics. 2007;33:308-10.

Spencer J. ABC's of Learning and teaching in medicine: learning and teaching in the clinical environment. BMJ. 2003;326:591-4.

Stevens DP, Holland GJ, Kizer KW. Results of a nationwide Veterans Affairs initiative to align graduate medical education and patient care. JAMA. 2001;286:1061-6.

Thorpe KE. Protecting the uninsured. N Engl J Med. 2004;351:1479-81.

Assessment, Feedback, Evaluation, Certification, and Licensing

Patrick C. Alguire, MD

Introduction	172
Feedback	172
Formative Feedback	172
Summative Feedback	173
Feedback Problems	173
Getting Better Feedback	173
Self-Assessment and Professional Development	174
The Feedback Sandwich	175
Barriers to Effective Feedback	176
Reflection	176
Evaluation	176
Basic Steps in the Evaluation Process	177
Assessment	177
Common Assessment Instruments	178
Other Assessment Systems	180
End-of-Rotation Evaluation	181
Retention, Promotion, and Dismissal	182
Licensure	183
Regulatory Paperwork	184
Certification	186

Introduction

This chapter addresses the relationship between assessment, feedback, and evaluation and ends with information about licensure and certification. *Assessment* is the process of collecting information about your performance. Assessment of knowledge, skills, and professionalism occurs throughout the medical career but is most formalized during residency training. *Feedback* is the process of telling you how you are performing in relation to established expectations (learning goals or competencies). *Evaluation* is simply assigning a grade (numerical, letter, or description) to your performance. During residency training, your evaluations will be used to make decisions related to retention and promotion or dismissal from the program. Successful completion of the residency program is a prerequisite for *certification* in your specialty, and successful progression through a number of years of the program is required to obtain a *license* to practice medicine in the United States.

Feedback

Feedback is an essential part of helping learners improve and is the most commonly cited "teaching" method described in the medical education literature. Ideally, it is based on first-hand assessment of a learner's knowledge, attitude, and skills. Expertly provided feedback describes actions or behaviors in such a way that it guides future learning and performance.

Despite the importance of feedback, the complaint heard most frequently from residents is that no one tells them how they are doing. As professionals, we do not make errors on purpose and most errors that persist are the result of insufficient feedback. Specific feedback is important because it has the potential to change our behavior in a positive direction. For example, intensive feedback provided to residents significantly improves satisfaction ratings from patients as compared with residents not receiving feedback. Ideally, feedback should be provided with every learning encounter, but realistically this is seldom possible. The minimal expectation is to receive feedback at regular intervals.

FORMATIVE FEEDBACK

Two different types of feedback are commonly used; brief (formative) feedback and formal (summative) feedback. Brief feedback is the kind you might receive after listening for a carotid bruit or following a case presentation during teaching rounds. It is spontaneous, short, and to the point. Here are two examples: "This is how I listen for a carotid bruit" and "Remember to begin your presentations with the patient's name, age, and reason why she is being seen today." If this advice is introduced with the statement, "Let me give you some feedback", it is easy to recognize as feedback. Often however, feedback is not identified so clearly and its full importance is lost. As a resident physician, you must increase your sensitivity to this type of feedback because your attending physician will expect you to internalize it and change your behavior accordingly. Failure to recognize brief feedback and follow through with the required behavior change will result in a poor evaluation. If the feedback message is not clear or you are unsure how to proceed, ask for clarification. Nothing is more gratifying to an attending physician than a resident responding positively to feedback by showing interest and a willingness to change; this too will be reflected in your evaluation, but as a positive attribute.

SUMMATIVE FEEDBACK

Formal (summative) feedback takes place at a planned feedback session, often scheduled at the middle and end of clinical rotations. Mid-rotation feedback allows you to "change course" before the rotation has ended. If you are not meeting the faculty's expectations, mid-rotation is the time to find out so you can improve before the rotation's end. Not all training programs mandate a mid-rotation evaluation session, but when offered, it should signal the need for change and improvement. Most training programs mandate or encourage end of rotation feedback during which the attending physician summarizes your performance and outlines "next steps" for you. This type of formal feedback and evaluation may take from 5 to 20 minutes and is usually documented, shared with the program director, and stored in your permanent evaluation file.

FEEDBACK PROBLEMS

Many attending physicians find it hard to give critical feedback. One reason is role conflict. Attending physicians see themselves as an advocate—a person helping residents succeed—, but at the same time attending physicians must ensure good patient care and maintain the standards of the profession. With these divided loyalties, attending physicians are often hesitant to give critical feedback, fearing loss of their helping, advocacy role. Another reason feedback is not provided as often as it should is that quality feedback is time consuming to plan, execute, and document. As a result, the pressures of patient care and other duties are often given higher priority than feedback. For many attending physicians, giving feedback, particularly if it is critical, is emotionally draining and difficult to do, particularly if the attending physician has emotionally bonded with the residents under his or her supervision. Finally, some teachers just are not skilled at providing quality feedback, often because of lack of training, but you can help them do a better job.

GETTING BETTER FEEDBACK

It is possible and even desirable to take an active role in your medical education. One area that is often neglected by learners is to engage their attending physician in a dialog related to their self-improvement. For example, by using a few simple strategies you can successfully set expectations for more frequent feedback, extract feedback that is timely, specific, and actionable, and have the attending physician prioritize the content of feedback.

Feedback that is expected and acted upon by the learner encourages the attending physician to provide additional feedback. You can politely and respectfully set the expectation for feedback by periodically asking for it. Learn to recognize natural feedback opportunities and use the opportunities to inquire about your performance. Such opportunities often crop up immediately after examining a patient in front of the attending physician, completing a case presentation, or following a night on call. By asking about your performance you benefit in several ways. The most obvious benefit is the feedback you receive to improve future performance. Also, by asking for feedback, you demonstrate a highly developed sense of professionalism and interest in improving, thereby setting an expectation of receiving additional feedback in the future. This is highly recommended strategy to get the most out of your training experience.

Learners get the most from feedback when it is timely, provided as close to the incident event as possible, and when it is specific. For example, don't ask for feedback on a cardiac examination you performed last week but rather get the feedback as close to when you performed the exam as possible so both you and the attending physician can remember what took place. As a learner, don't be satisfied with general praise or criticism but gently push the attending for more detailed information. If told, "You did a good job on that cardiac examination" you should ask, "What aspects should I continue to do and what should I improve?" Similarly, if you are told, "That cardiac exam was not complete," ask "How can I do it better?" or "Can you show me how to do it?"

Sometimes the amount of feedback you can get is overwhelming. In these situations it is hard to know what is important and what can be put off until later, or even the most logical order to address the deficiencies. Being overwhelmed with information impedes your ability to identify and focus on the negative behaviors that might be holding you back. For example, you might be told, "You don't seem to know when to initiate insulin therapy, how to monitor therapy, current therapeutic goals for diabetes, or how to follow up on treatment. You also lack confidence when talking with patients and give confusing instructions, and your notes are disorganized." This is a lot of information and it all sounds important, but it is too much for any learner to act upon. If this happens, ask the attending physician for clarification. The most effective strategy is to ask him or her which two or three items need to be worked on first and for some suggestions for making improvements in those areas. This is an important point; not only is it the attending physician's responsibility to provide timely and specific feedback, but there is also a responsibility to help you improve. This might take the form of personal instruction, arranging for others to help, or referring you to independent study resources. Using this strategy you should be able to get concrete information on what to do next. You might be told, "Read this chapter on starting insulin therapy, and be prepared to discuss it with me tomorrow morning." While this does not address all of the learning problems identified by the attending physician, it is a first step that is both practical and logical and avoids your having to guess what to do next.

Good feedback addresses behaviors that you can control. You may sometimes receive feedback about which you can do nothing, and it is important to recognize this when it occurs. For example, an attending physician may comment, "Your accent is so pronounced that no one understands you." Since it is unlikely that you will change your accent in the near future, you need a strategy to identify what you can do to address the underlying problem. Begin by analyzing the problem and reflecting on its importance. In this example, the criticism relates to your communication skills. Begin your dialog with the attending physician by acknowledging the legitimacy of his/her criticism, that you are concerned about it, and that you want to take action. For example, you might say, "I understand that I need to communicate better with my patients but I don't think I can change my accent very quickly. Do you have any advice for me?" After some reflection, the attending physician might recommend that you speak more slowly, or frequently stop and check with the patient for understanding. Both these behaviors you can do and are likely to result in improvement. The attending physician will be impressed with your professional attitude and willingness to make changes.

SELF-ASSESSMENT AND PROFESSIONAL DEVELOPMENT

Many experienced attending physicians begin a feedback session by asking for your own self-assessment. You might be asked, "What went well and what could you have done better?" A question like this is often asked to judge your own insight into your performance (both good and bad) and is a jumping-off point for the delivery of high-quality feedback. It is much easier to provide specific feedback if both the teacher and learner agree on the problem and almost impossible to provide effective feedback if they do not. If both you and the attending physician agree that your greatest strength is your charismatic personality and ability to get along with others but your cardiac examination is weak, this meeting of the minds facilitates an open and honest conversation on improving the cardiac examination. Therefore this is the time to be brutally honest. The candid use of self-assessment promotes a professional dialog between you and the attending physician and facilitates the exchange of higher quality, more specific information.

THE FEEDBACK SANDWICH

Many educators use some variation of the "feedback sandwich" for both formal and brief feedback. The "feedback sandwich" comprises three components delivered in the following order:

- What was done right
- What was done wrong
- What to do next time

A feedback sandwich might be delivered to you like this: "I like the way you examined the heart. You were methodical, going through each step of inspection, palpation, percussion, and auscultation. However, I noticed that you used only the diaphragm of the stethoscope and not the bell. The bell is important when listening for low-pitched sounds. On subsequent patients, I want you to listen with the bell at each major area. This will allow you to better hear the low-pitched sounds." It is important to recognize the feedback sandwich for what it is: feedback. As feedback, there is an expectation that you will act on the information. It is important to pay attention to the entire "sandwich." Understand that the praise part of the feedback sandwich (*what was done right*) is a strong signal to continue with the behavior that earned the praise. This behavior is valued by the attending physician and needs to become routine. The "meat" of the sandwich (*what was done wrong*) contains the improvement message; this is what you need to work on. Listen carefully to the last part of the sandwich (*what to do next time*) because it contains detailed instructions for improvement and often suggestions for practice. At this point, it is customary for the attending physician to ask for your comments. Use this opportunity to clarify the nature of the deficiency by gathering as much specific information as possible. Summarize what you have heard and what you need to do next; this is a great strategy that demonstrates professionalism and validates what needs to be done next. Convey a willingness to act on what you have heard and even suggest a follow-up meeting to check on your progress. These actions show that you are ready to take the next steps to meet the attending physician's expectations.

To summarize, feedback is part of learning and is most effective if you take an active role in the process. Ask for feedback throughout the learning experience by learning to recognize feedback opportunities, then act upon them. Select an appropriate time and place (often private) as soon as possible after the learning event. Prevent feedback overload by asking the attending physician to select one or two important behaviors for you to work on. Recognize the value of self-assessment and the feedback sandwich and use both to engage your attending physician in a dialog about your performance and how to improve it.

BARRIERS TO EFFECTIVE FEEDBACK

There are two important barriers to effective feedback. The first barrier is the attending physician. If the attending physician does not take the time, or is insecure, or simply unskilled in providing feedback, feedback will not be effective. The previous section discusses strategies to engage the attending physician in ways to improve the quantity and quality of the feedback. The second barrier is how you receive the feedback. No one can honestly say that they enjoy criticism, or that it doesn't hurt to hear that improvement is needed. Despite this, it is incumbent upon you to act in a professional manner. See Box 9-1 for some important "do's and don'ts" to remember when receiving feedback.

☑ **BOX 9-1** **"Do's and Don'ts" When Receiving Feedback**

■ *Do* listen attentively.
■ *Do* ask appropriate questions to clarify or add specificity.
■ *Do* ask about next steps or advice on how to improve.
■ *Do* offer thanks for the feedback.
■ *Do* make the effort to follow-through.

■ *Don't* argue or contradict.
■ *Don't* ignore advice or minimize its importance.
■ *Don't* assume that just because this is the first time you have been criticized that the criticism is not valid. ("No one has ever said this to me before; therefore it must be wrong.")

REFLECTION

In the context of professional practice, reflection is essential in the educational experience for learners. For many learners, reflection after receiving feedback provides the impetus for change and improvement. Assessing what went well and what went wrong are key steps in this process. In the feedback process, personal reflection usually takes place after receiving feedback when you had time to think about what was said. Review in your mind what was said about your performance. What did you do well? Why was this singled out? Do you agree? What wasn't done well? Why was this brought up? Why is it important? What can I do to get better? What will I need to get better?

Excellent residents use this information to make important improvements, and this represents the pinnacle of professionalism; mediocre residents never change or even consider the need to change. The American Board of Internal Medicine has developed an evaluation tool for resident self-evaluation and reflection (http://www.abim.org/pdf/papertools/Residents_Competency.pdf) and is a useful guide to this important process.

Evaluation

It is sometimes difficult to understand the difference between feedback and evaluation. Evaluation assigns a numerical or descriptive "value" to your performance. The value is typically judged against goals established for the learning experience by the residency program. As such, most residents equate evaluation with receiving a score at the end of the rotation. Accordingly, this section addresses aspects of the end-of-rotation and semi-annual evaluations.

Typically, residency programs collect summative evaluations from faculty to meet the following educational needs:

- Determining learner competence and identifying learner strengths and weaknesses
- Identifying strengths and weaknesses of the curriculum
- Making decisions about retention and promotion
- Providing information to outside institutions (e.g., for fellowship or employment positions)
- Maintaining accreditation of the institution
- Providing legal documentation

BASIC STEPS IN THE EVALUATION PROCESS

All training programs must create a set of learning goals and objectives or competencies that are to be mastered by the resident prior to graduation. Most institutions list these desired knowledge, attitudinal, and skill competencies on the evaluation form. An example of a prototypic evaluation form developed by the American Board of Internal Medicine (ABIM) for internal medicine residency programs is available online (http://www.abim.org/pdf/paper-tools/AttendigCompetency.pdf). In this example, an evaluation rating scale measures the degree to which the learner mastered the competencies. This is usually the "gold standard" against which your progress is measured in the training program.

Regardless of the specialty training program, there are basic evaluation steps common to all. The first step is assessment which consists of gathering performance data from a variety of sources that informs the evaluation decision. The second step is a meeting of the resident and attending physician at the end of the rotation to review overall performance and receive formal (summative) feedback. The third step is completed when the attending physician (and sometimes others, described below) documents his/her evaluation and submits it to the program director. The final step requires that all residents meet with the program director, usually twice per year, to review the new evaluations in their evaluation portfolio and to receive counseling and guidance.

ASSESSMENT

It is a good idea to review the standard rotation evaluation form at the beginning of training. Most residency training programs will provide you with a copy during orientation, or you can obtain a copy from the residency administration office. The evaluation form is a succinct document which in part functions to "communicate" the basic goals of the experience and records how well you are meeting the goals. Faculty may use a variety of data sources on your performance to fill out the form (Box 9-2).

☑ **BOX 9-2 Data Sources for Assessment Form**

- Direct observation of performance during rounds or in the clinic
- Review of written records (e.g., progress notes, history, physical examination findings)
- Oral case presentations
- Responses to questions
- Interactions with clinic or hospital staff
- Patient comments or measures of satisfaction
- Your self-evaluation

The most reliable method of collecting performance data is direct observation (e.g., watching you take a history, perform an examination or procedure, or counsel a patient). A very popular assessment method, the mini-clinical evaluation exercise (mini-CEX), has been developed by the ABIM and has been adopted by a number of other specialties. This exercise focuses on assessing core skills that residents can demonstrate during their daily encounters with patients. Specifically, the mini-CEX is a 15 to 20 minute faculty observation of a resident-patient encounter. When performed repeatedly over time with multiple patients, this exercise provides a valid and reliable assessment of a resident's performance. The mini-CEX evaluation form can be obtained from the ABIM Web site at (http://www.abim.org/pdf/paper-tools/minicex.pdf).

Other tried-and-true methods include how you respond to questions about your patients. Can you generate a logical differential diagnosis (or treatment plan) and prioritize it from most to least likely diagnosis (or best treatment)? Can you defend your choices with data collected from the history, physical, and laboratory evaluation? Observing how you interact with other members of the hospital or clinic staff and soliciting their opinion of you is another important source of evaluation data. Patients are another good source of primary data, and their comments are often collected formally (by asking them to fill out a written survey) or informally (by staff asking casual questions).

COMMON ASSESSMENT INSTRUMENTS

The common requirements for residency programs mandate that residency programs collect evaluation data on residents from multiple sources. To help fill this evaluation need, the Accreditation Council for Graduate Medical Education and the American Board of Medical Specialties have created a list of potential evaluation tools for residency programs. In addition to the faculty evaluation form (discussed above), a residency program is required to use one or more than one of these tools. For the purposes of this chapter, this list has been modified and reproduced below to provide an overview of evaluation methodologies you may encounter during residency training. For a more in-depth description of these evaluation tools, visit the ACGME Web site (http://www.acgme.org/Outcome/assess/Toolbox.pdf). The ratings from these evaluation tools are typically summarized for all evaluators, reviewed by the program director, and filed into your evaluation folder.

360-Degree Evaluation

This evaluation is completed by multiple people in the resident's immediate environment (e.g., faculty, peers, subordinates, nurses, administration staff, patients and families). Most tools of this nature use a survey or questionnaire to gather information on your performance in several areas (e.g., teamwork, communication, management skills, decision-making) using a rating scale to assess how frequently a desired behavior is performed. The importance of this evaluation methodology is to recognize that you may be evaluated by non-physician staff and that you should accord these professionals the same courtesy and respect of an attending physician.

Chart Stimulated Recall

A chart stimulated recall (CSR) examination involves reviewing several of your patient cases using a standardized oral examination technique. A trained and experienced physician examiner asks probing questions behind the work-up, diagnoses, interpretation of clinical findings, and treatment plans that are documented in a patient note that you generated. Often, you are allowed to pick the cases to be examined on. Each patient case takes 5 to 10 minutes, and three to six cases may be reviewed.

Checklists

Checklists consist of a list of essential or desired behaviors or steps that make up a more complex competency. The form is completed by simply indicating whether a step was completed or not and how well it was completed. Checklists are used to assess a variety of performances that have discrete recognizable components that must be performed in a logical sequence (e.g., physical examination maneuvers or procedural skills).

Objective Structured Clinical Examination

In an objective structured clinical examination (OSCE), you participate in 12 to 20 separate standardized patient encounters called *stations*, and each station lasts about 10-15 minutes. Standardized patients are professionally trained people who portray (simulate) different medical conditions. You are asked to examine the standardized patient as if he/she were a real patient. At the end of each encounter, you are asked to complete a patient note or other brief written description of the encounter. The evaluation of the encounter may include either observation by a faculty member or by the standardized patient using a checklist evaluation form. Although standardized patients are usually the primary assessment tool, some programs create OSCE encounters that require you to interpret data (e.g., chest x-ray, electrocardiogram, laboratory tests) or to use a mannequin to assess technical skills.

Logs

Procedure, operative, or case logs document your encounters with patients, surgical operations, or procedures. The logs often include counts of cases, operations, or procedures. Logs are typically used to document exposure to important conditions or procedures within a medical specialty. Logs vary in their detail with some logs recording only type of encounter and others recording more extensive data such as complications, patient outcomes, interpretation of findings, and written assessments by supervisors.

Patient Surveys

Surveys of patients are used to assess satisfaction with your care including amount of time spent with the patient, overall quality of care, physician competency, courtesy, and interest or empathy. A survey asks patients to rate their satisfaction with care using rating categories or agreement with statements describing the care.

Portfolio

A portfolio is a collection of products prepared by the resident that provides evidence of learning. A portfolio typically contains written documents but can include video- or audio-recordings, photographs, and other forms of information. A written essay reflecting upon what has been learned is often included in a portfolio. A typical portfolio may include a log of procedures performed, a written case report or other scholarly activity, a quality improvement project plan, or a recording or transcript of counseling provided to patients.

Simulations and Models

Simulations are used for assessment of clinical performance by closely imitating a clinical encounter. Most commonly used simulations use computer models (virtual colonoscopy or bronchoscopy), mannequins (cardiac arrest, central line placement, arthrocentesis), recordings (heart sounds, breath sounds), or standardized patients (patient education and counseling).

Written Examination (In-Training Examination)

A written or computer-based multiple-choice question (MCQ) examination assesses medical knowledge. Typically, the examination is clinically-based, with each question presented as a short case scenario followed by four or five potential answers. The most popular of these examinations are the "in-training" examinations prepared by specialty societies and certifying boards and take half to a full day to complete. Most in-training examinations are offered during the second year of a three-year training program and compare your performance on the examination to all other residents in the United States taking the same examination. Examinations of this type have excellent predictive capability for performance on the specialty board certifying examination taken at the end of residency training. The results of the in-training examination are typically used to counsel residents who, based upon their examination score, are in danger of not passing the certifying examination. These examinations are not used to determine promotion or retention within the residency program.

OTHER ASSESSMENT SYSTEMS

The RIME evaluation system is another commonly used assessment system. RIME is a mnemonic for a set of progressively complex and sophisticated clinical skills. Many physicians prefer to use the RIME evaluation method because it is easy to remember, intuitive to use, and requires no special forms or tools. Furthermore, the RIME system focuses on the traditional core skills that need to be mastered by a resident in any specialty area. The components of the RIME system are given in Box 9-3.

☑ BOX 9-3 **RIME Evaluation System**

- **R**eporter: Consistently collects and reports data in an accurate, organized way.
- **I**nterpreter: Consistently interprets history clues, physical-examination findings, and laboratory results; creates and prioritizes problem lists and creates and justifies a differential diagnosis.
- **M**anager: Consistently selects and applies appropriate diagnostic and treatment options that best meet the patient's needs.
- **E**ducator: Identifies and addresses knowledge gaps using evidence-based approaches; educates the patient and colleagues using his or her knowledge, clinical reasoning, and analytic skills.

Each step in the RIME model represents a synthesis of knowledge, attitude, and skill that is practiced and mastered as a learner progresses from the preclinical years of medical school through residency training, reflecting the transitions from a novice to an expert clinician. Mastering each level depends on mastering the previous level. RIME is also useful because it is a much more reliable way to evaluate a learner's skills. Each faculty member who has been trained to use the RIME evaluation framework can "reliably" evaluate learners' skills (the ability to get the same results as other faculty members).

The RIME framework also has strong predictive validity; in other words, the result predicts future performance, such as on the end of clerkship examination for medical students. It is valuable for you to know about the RIME evaluation system so you can appreciate how you might be evaluated by faculty. This will allow you to focus on and improve on skills central to the evaluation scheme.

A "Reporter" can efficiently and accurately collect history and physical-examination data, can recognize normal and abnormal findings, and can identify and label new problems. Additionally, a reporter is capable of communicating this information orally and in writing in an organized way. Mastery of skills at the reporter level is expected of all third-year students. Mastery of "Interpreter" skills means that the learner interprets data, develops a differential diagnosis, prioritizes problems and differential diagnoses from most likely to least likely, and follows up on and interprets results of physical findings and diagnostic tests. Mastery of this skill level is expected of senior medical students and interns (first-year residents). "Managers" are capable of determining when action is necessary (versus "watchful waiting"), select the best diagnostic and therapeutic options, and customize care according to patient circumstances and preferences. They take the initiative to search out answers and alternatives to clinical questions. Mastery at the manager level requires advanced knowledge, confidence, clinical reasoning and judgment, and is most often attained by junior and senior (second- and third-year) residents. An "Educator" is capable of identifying knowledge gaps and takes the initiative to address these gaps. Educators synthesize and share new knowledge with others and understand the uses and limitations of evidence in the care of patients. These skills take drive, insight, and maturity and are most likely to be present in senior residents and practitioners.

END-OF-ROTATION EVALUATION

The common requirements for all residency training programs stipulate that faculty must evaluate resident performance in a timely manner during each rotation or similar educational assignment, and document this evaluation at completion of the assignment. To complete this task, a time is usually set aside by the faculty to review in private your evaluation before it is returned to the program director. You may be asked to fill out a copy of the evaluation before this meeting as a self-evaluation exercise. This sets the stage for the upcoming discussion with the faculty that will focus on your strengths and areas of needed improvement. Additionally, the self-evaluation process provides you with an opportunity to reflect on your performance, a professional behavior expected of physicians in the "real world".

During this meeting you are likely to receive some final feedback, which if done skillfully will include examples of behaviors that support the final evaluation. You may be asked to sign the evaluation report at the end of the session, indicating you reviewed it with the attending physician. Your signature does not imply that you agree with the evaluation, only that you have reviewed it. If you do not agree with the evaluation, there are processes and procedures built into the residency program that will allow you to address your concerns.

During the end of rotation evaluation, the attending physician may solicit your comments about the experience, including you thoughts on the teaching process. Most residents are reluctant to discuss their opinions with the attending physician at this time, but other avenues are available for you to comment on the educational process. To maintain compliance with the common accreditation guidelines, all residency programs must, at least annually, evaluate faculty performance as it relates to the educational program. These evaluations should include a review of the faculty's clinical teaching abilities, commitment to the educational program, clinical knowledge, professionalism, and scholarly activities. This evaluation must include at least annual written confidential evaluations by the residents. In keeping with these guidelines, the program director will provide you with an opportunity to evaluate the experience and the attending physician. The aggregated (an anonymous) results from many residents over time are provided to the attending physician to improve his/her teaching.

RETENTION, PROMOTION, AND DISMISSAL

The common accreditation requirements for residency programs provide very clear direction as it relates to resident retention, promotion, and graduation. Faculty are required to provide objective assessments of your competence in the six ACGME core competencies of patient care, medical knowledge, practice-based learning and improvement, interpersonal and communication skills, professionalism, and systems-based practice. Residency training programs are required to use multiple evaluators (e.g., faculty, peers, patients, self, other professional staff) to document your progression through the training program and take special care to document that your improvement is continuous and appropriate to your educational level. Finally, the program director is required to meet with you for a semiannual evaluation of your performance and to review your evaluations since the last meeting. Most program directors will take this opportunity and provide feedback, counseling, and career guidance. The feedback will focus on your progression through the training program with particular attention to whether you are "on course" (ability appropriate for level of training) or in academic difficulty. In the vast majority of cases, residents are told that they are progressing satisfactorily, but this is not always the case. For residents experiencing academic difficulty, the program director must tell the resident the nature of the deficiency and the consequences of the resident's failure to adequately remediate the deficiency.

Residency programs can dismiss residents, not renew contracts, or not promote to the next training year for failure related to academic progress or professionalism. It is the collective judgment of the faculty as to whether a resident is making satisfactory progress in the training program and faculty have absolute broad discretion in determining whether a resident is academically or professionally delinquent. If a dismissal or promotion decision is contested in a court of law, the burden of proof is on the resident to prove that he or she met the academic standard or was treated in an arbitrary and capricious manner (i.e., a decision not based upon facts or a decision that is intentionally malicious). Non-cognitive factors are an important part of academic performance and thus grounds for dismissal. Personal hygiene, ability to get along with peers and faculty, and punctuality may be as important factors in a program's decision of whether a resident will make a good medical doctor as is the ability to take a case history or diagnose an illness. Residents can also be dismissed because they violated an institutional rule or regulation. In these special and somewhat unusual circumstances, the burden of proof lies with the program to demonstrate that the resident did violate the rules or regulations. In this case, formal hearings are required, rules of evidentiary evidence take precedence (similar to those used in a court of law), and strict attention to due process must be maintained.

In instances where a resident's contract will not be renewed, or when a resident will not be promoted to the next level of training, the institution sponsoring the training program must provide the resident with a written notice of this intent no later than four months prior to the end of the current agreement. If the primary reason for the nonrenewal or non-promotion occurs within the four months prior to the end of the current agreement, the institution must provide the resident with as much written notice of the intent not to renew or not to promote as circumstances will reasonably allow, prior to the end of the agreement.

Residents faced with academic dismissal, nonrenewal, or failure of promotion have limited recourse. According to the common accreditation guidelines, residents must be allowed to implement the institution's grievance procedures if they receive a written notice of either intent not to renew their agreement or not to promote to the next level of training. An institution's grievance procedure must be based upon a written set of policies and procedures that allow a resident to present arguments against nonrenewal, dismissal, or failure of promotion. Most institutional grievance procedures have in common three components. The resident

1. Must receive notice of his or her deficiencies
2. Have an opportunity to examine the evaluations
3. Should be allowed to present his or her side of the story to the decision-maker (usually the program director or chairman of the department).

However, institutional grievance procedures are not required to mandate formal hearings or even face-to-face dialog between the resident and the decision-maker (e.g., arguments may be presented in writing). Furthermore, residents do not have the right to be represented by legal counsel (e.g., a lawyer). Adverse decisions do not require faculty unanimity or even consensus support; the residency program is not required to treat all dismissal and promotion cases the same, even if circumstances are similar; and requirements for retention and promotion do not have to be uniformly applied to all residents, provided there is a documented and reasoned rationale for altering the requirements. These points underscore the wide discretionary powers enjoyed by residency programs when judging the academic progress and professionalism of residents.

Licensure

Physicians in the United States are licensed to practice medicine by individual state medical boards. In addition, State medical boards investigate complaints, and discipline those who violate the law. State medical boards are typically made up of volunteer physicians and members of the public. A medical license is state specific and physicians must apply for a new medical license in each state in which they intend to practice. Your residency program will assist you in obtaining a restricted medical license for training purposes, but if you plan to stay in the United States to practice medicine, you will be solely responsible for obtaining the permanent medical license. Be aware that hospital credentialing and qualification for medical malpractice insurance are processes that can begin only after you are in possession of a full and unrestricted medical license. Because all of these steps take considerable time to complete, begin the process as early as possible to ensure that you can actually begin to practice medicine when you need to. A handy resource for up-to-date information on state licensure, including licensing requirements, fees, license renewal, and continuing medical education, is the American Medical

Association's *State Medical License Requirements and Statistics* (available for purchase in both print and electronic formats; 1-800-621-8335).

In order to be licensed you must meet state-specific requirements. Requirements common to all states for initial licensure include a medical degree, possession of a valid certificate from the ECFMG, passage of all the USMLE licensing examination steps, and meeting all requirements imposed by the individual state licensing authority. In general, state licensing requirements require a minimum number of postgraduate (residency) training years (typically more for international medical graduates compared to US medical graduates) and a requirement to complete the USMLE process within a specified period of time. The specific state requirements can be reviewed on the Federation of State Medical Boards Web site (http://www.fsmb.org/usmle_eliinitial.html).

Regulatory Paperwork

For a smooth transition from residency or fellowship training to practice, you must pay attention to the paperwork. The paperwork must be done in a timely fashion and be meticulously complete to avoid delays in beginning your clinical practice. The medical license application process may take between 4 to 6 months but is sometimes longer for international medical graduates. Be aware that the highest volume of licensure applications is received between the months of April and September, when physicians with families begin the relocation process before the academic school year for their children and resident physicians traditionally begin the application process. Applications can be obtained by writing or calling the state licensing agency. Many state medical boards provide information about the application process and allow you to download the appropriate application through the Internet (www.fsmb.org/).

Although state licensing board requirements vary, they generally request the same types of core information, including a notarized personal photograph of the applicant, medical school transcripts, a copy of the medical diploma, USMLE scores, ECFMG certificate, documentation of postgraduate training, and a report from the National Practitioner Data Bank (NPDM). The NPDB [http://www.npdb-hipdb.com/welcomesq.html] is a repository of adverse actions taken against physicians including malpractice claims or settlements, state medical board sanctions, convictions for fraud or abuse, and other similar data. Many state Boards also reference the Federation of State Medical Boards (FSMB) Physician Data Center (http://www.fsmb.org/m_fpdc.html), which contains similar information. A physician should never try to hide derogatory information from a licensing board or provide information that is less than complete. It is much better to come forward with the information and assist the board in obtaining records and other necessary information, and provide information about mitigating circumstances that might prevent license denial. Some state licensing boards may request a resume or curriculum vitae or may require a personal appearance. These allow the licensing board to evaluate your application for potential problems early in the process and will give you advance notice of any extra steps or delays that might arise. In the resource area of this book is information on how to write a resume and construct a curriculum vitae.

Many state medical boards also request your curriculum vitae. It is important that the dates on your curriculum vitae correspond exactly to the dates from the various institutions documenting your training, and that there be no unexplained gaps of time. The medical license application will be very specific as to how the required information should be accessed, and how it should be transmitted to the licensing agency. Failure to follow the application instructions precisely will result in long and costly delays. It is advisable when beginning the application process to create an organizational chart that details what information you have requested, when it was requested, to whom the request was sent (name, address and telephone number), and a notation of any processing fee that was sent (check number and date). Your requests for documentation from the various organizations must be made in writing, and you should always make a copy of your correspondence for future reference.

It is not unusual to discover that your application has been delayed because an institution (a medical school, for example) did not forward the needed information to the licensing agency as requested. It is your responsibility, not the responsibility of the licensing agency, to contact the wayward institution and follow up on the missing documentation. When making calls to the institution, always take down the full name and title of the person helping you, and put that information on your organizational chart for future reference. Finally, it is a good idea to contact the licensing agency periodically (e.g., every 6 weeks) to check on the progress of your application. Do not rely on the licensing agency to inform you of missing or incomplete information.

As a service to physicians, the Federation of State Medical Boards offers a Credentials Verification Service (FCVS) [http://www.fsmb.org/fcvs.html]. For a fee, the CVS will obtain primary source verification from the entity that issued them of the credentials most commonly needed for a medical license, including verification of your identity, medical school transcripts, postgraduate training, USMLE or other licensing examination record, and ECFMG certification. Importantly, the FCVS has collaborated with the Educational Commission for Foreign Medical Graduates (ECFMG) to reduce the duplication of efforts and redundancy in primary source verification of medical diplomas and transcripts for international medical school graduates. Physician applicants to FCVS need to complete the ECFMG Release forms (included in the FCVS on-line application or paper application on the FCVS web site) and FCVS will coordinate with ECFMG to verify the physician's medical education credentials. Subsequent profiles can be forwarded to other recipients (e.g., other state medical boards, insurance plans, hospital-credentialing committees) for a fee. Despite the expense, there are several potential advantages to the FCVS, not the least being the amount of time this service can save you. In addition, all state boards accept FCVS services and some actually require them. Once FCVS has completed the initial application process, it maintains a permanent record of all your primary documents for future use and provides the peace of mind of having these important documents securely stored.

Other important paperwork includes obtaining your insurance provider numbers. In order to be paid by third party insurance carriers, you must have a provider number for each insurance company and managed care organization with which you wish to participate. If you are joining another physician or group, chances are the office staff will obtain these numbers for you. If you have previously moonlighted (worked as a physician outside of the residency program), you may already have your Medicare provider number; this federal identification number never changes once it is assigned to you. The State Survey Agency (http://www.cms.hhs.gov/MedicareProviderSupEnroll/) most often supplies the Medicare and Medicaid provider numbers to new physicians.

Physicians who prescribe controlled substances will need a Drug Enforcement Agency (DEA) Controlled Substance Registration Certificate. An application can be obtained by calling 1-800-882-9539 or going to http://www.deadiversion.usdoj.gov/drugreg/index.html.

Some states also require a State Controlled Substance License. This application is usually part of the state medical license application.

If you are beginning your own practice, you may be required to obtain a Federal Employee Identification Number (FEIN) (http://www.irs.gov/businesses/small/article/0,,id=102767,00.html).

The FEIN is required of any business that takes tax and other payroll deductions from the salary of one or more employees, and is obtained by filling out IRS form SS-4. A different number is required for each unique site of business. If joining a group or organization, you will not need to obtain a FEIN, because it is site specific, not person specific. Many states and cities also mandate a State Employee Identification Number, and this is usually obtained from the respective departments of treasury. Like the FEIN, the state number is business, not person specific.

The Health Care Financing Agency regulates all laboratory testing through the Clinical Laboratory Improvement Amendments (CLIA) (http://www.cms.hhs.gov/clia/) program. For offices that perform even minor laboratory tests, a CLIA certificate is required. If starting a practice, you must apply for certification; if joining a practice or organization, the certification will already be in place. Like the FEIN, the CLIA certification is site, not person, specific.

Certification

Medical specialty certification in the United States differs from licensure in that certification is a voluntary process. Medical licensure sets the minimum competency requirements to diagnose and treat patients but it is not specialty specific. Certification demonstrates that physicians have met vigorous standards through intensive study, self-assessment and evaluation, and demonstrates to the public expertise in a particular specialty and/or subspecialty of medical practice. Although each specialty and subspecialty sets its own standards for certification, there are a few common principles: a medical school diploma, satisfactory completion of residency and fellowship training requirements, meeting all state licensure requirements, and passing a certification examination. At one time, physicians were awarded certificates that were not time-limited and therefore did not have to be renewed. In 2006, all specialty boards adopted a new gold standard for re-certification called "Maintenance of Certification" (MOC). MOC requires proof of continuing education and other experiences in between testing for re-certification. The MOC cycle varies according to the specialty but ranges from 6 to 10 years. For detailed information on any specialty or subspecialty certification and maintenance of certification process, contact the American Board of Medical Specialties at http://www.abms.org/About_Board_Certification/.

Living in America: Popular Culture

Gerald P. Whelan, MD

Introduction	188
Finding a Place to Live	188
Day-to-Day Living	189
Obtaining Necessary Items	189
■ Social Security Card	189
■ Driver's License	190
Getting Settled	191
Bank Accounts and Credit Cards	191
■ Bank Accounts	191
■ Credit Cards	192
Food	193
Transportation	194
Personal Health Care	195
Religious Activities	195
Recreational Activities	196
Individual Activities	196
Group Activities and Meeting People	196
Travel	197
Family Considerations	197
Should Spouse/Family Accompany the IMG?	197
Spouse Employment/Educational Options	198
Schools	198
Emergency Assistance	199
Getting Local Information	199

Introduction

Although training in a residency or fellowship can be quite demanding in terms of time and energy, life can and must go on outside of the hospital and the training program. To function well as a physician and to maximize learning as a student, it is critical to be well rested, in good mental and physical health, and periodically have some recreation. For IMGs who are accompanied by spouses and/or family, it is necessary to balance the demands of training programs with the need to pay attention to personal relationships and the desires and needs of family members. This section provides some practical information on living in the United States and understanding its popular culture.

Finding a Place to Live

Perhaps the most critical order of business when beginning a training program, after ensuring that all necessary paperwork and requirements with respect to the program have been taken care of, is finding a suitable place to live.

Hospital dormitories do exist but are not as prevalent as they were in past years. If they are available, they tend to be fairly minimalist and generally provide only a single or shared room. Bathroom facilities may be private or shared, and cooking and refrigeration facilities are quite variable. There will likely be some common areas with television, music systems, and reading areas, and there may be access to fitness facilities. Dormitories are generally not appropriate for spouses and/or children, and they are less than ideal as a long-term living arrangement. All hospitals have "call rooms" where residents can sleep while on call overnight in the hospital, and these may be located in dormitories.

A significant step-up from dormitories are hospital- or institution-owned and operated apartments or townhouses. These are generally comfortable and well-maintained and usually offered at a reasonable rate. They may not be as spacious as commercially available properties but are probably adequate for a physician and spouse and in some cases small children. Larger families or families with older children may find them somewhat constraining. These units have private bathroom facilities and fully equipped kitchens, usually have landline telephones, and are generally furnished, although occupants may need to provide their own televisions, music systems, and other personal equipment.

Because availability of hospital or institution dormitories or other housing is so variable, information must be obtained directly from the training program. In some cases such accommodations may be available when trainees first arrive, but there may be limits on how long they can continue to occupy them. Arrangements like these may also be useful while the new resident fellow is searching for more long-term accommodations.

The most common initial living arrangement for most newly arriving IMGs is a rented apartment or house. Many programs may have lists of rental properties or referrals to real estate agents, and this should probably be the first place to begin.

In choosing a rental property, there are several issues to consider. Because the resident will be spending a great deal of time at the hospital and commuting back and forth, the property should be relatively nearby the hospital or at least convenient to roadways and/or public transportation. In addition to proximity, residents should consider the quality of life and safety of a neighborhood. Certain areas may have particularly high crime rates and may be dangerous for residents or fellows coming or going late at night. The safety of the area is also a consideration with respect to spouses and children.

Program staff at the hospital, residents in the program, or advisors will generally be knowledgeable about the safety and desirability of neighborhoods and should definitely be consulted. In fact, one of the best questions to ask residents and staff in the program is "Where do you live?"

The size of a rental property is also subject to many factors. First is the number of occupants. A resident unaccompanied by a spouse or family may find it most practicable to share a rental property with one or more other single residents. Since each year some residents complete training and move on, it may be worthwhile trying to discover if someone in the training program, or even in other training programs, is looking for a new roommate. At the other extreme, a resident who is accompanied by a spouse and several children or other relatives may need a significantly bigger property with multiple bedrooms and bathrooms. Of course, the bigger the property, the higher the rent, so the amount of money available may be the final determining factor with respect to the size of the apartment or house that may be rented.

Renters will require evidence of a good credit history (see below) as well as evidence of employment. The latter can be provided by showing the program contract. It is also usual that the landlord will require the first month's rent plus an amount equal to an additional month or two of rent as security. This would be to cover any damage incurred to the property (if there is no damage, it should be returned on termination of the lease). The lease is the amount of time that the rental agreement is in effect. Some rentals are on a month-to-month basis; others will be on a single- or multiple-year basis. The longer lease ensures that the occupants will be able to stay in the property for the term of the lease, but it also makes it costly and difficult to move out of the property before the expiration of the lease.

Buying a house or other property on first arriving in the United States is probably not the wisest option. Aside from the expense, there is a great deal of paperwork involved, and in most cases it will be necessary to purchase through a real estate agent. Because many residents will be moving to a different area after completion of their training, it is probably best to defer buying a home until it is determined where one will be practicing in the long-term.

Day-to-Day Living

OBTAINING NECESSARY ITEMS

Two critical items for all newly arriving IMGs are a social security number (SSN) and a driver's license. The SSN is needed for several purposes. While not technically necessary to receive a salary, some institutions may withhold salary until a valid SSN is reported. It is also often required to open bank accounts or to get a credit card. Aside from the obvious purpose of allowing the holder to drive a motor vehicle, driver's licenses that contain photo identification are probably the most common form of identification used in daily activities in the United States.

Social Security Card

Laws and regulations regarding Social Security cards, driver's licenses, and related items are in a state of flux due to increasing and changing concerns about national security in the United States. Therefore the following information should be confirmed for accuracy and currency before definitively acting or planning to act on it.

Anyone, including accompanying persons such as spouses and other dependents, who will be earning money and therefore filing an income tax return (required by law) in the United States must have a valid SSN. However, the SSN application cannot be processed by the Social Security Administration until there is verification that the noncitizen has entered the country and reported to his or her employer or program. For IMGs on J-1 visas, this entails the program director notifying ECFMG of the resident's arrival and providing copies of travel documents and confirmation of employment start date. ECFMG then in turn reports this information to the Student Exchange Visa Information System (SEVIS) where it can then be accessed by the Social Security Administration. For those entering on other visas, their entry into the country initiates the notification process. In either case, in order to allow time for these steps to occur, the application process itself should not be started until at least 10 days after entry into the country. Applying before that time may actually increase the delay in obtaining a SSN.

The application form including detailed instructions can be downloaded from the Social Security Web site (www.socialsecurity.gov). It must be completed and submitted in person with the appropriate supporting documents at any local Social Security office. Their locations can be found on the Web site or via a toll-free telephone number (1-800-772-1213); this information may also be available from the program administrator. At the time of submission, all the original documents listed in Box 10-1 must be presented.

☑ BOX 10-1   **Documents Needed for Social Security Number Application**

■ Completed Application for Social Security Card (Form SS-5)
■ Valid I-94 card (Arrival/Departure Record) with accurate status dates
■ J-1 exchange visitors must also present a DS-2019 (Certificate of Eligibility for Exchange Visitor Status)
■ Original copy of the residency or fellowship contract signed by both the resident or fellow and the program director or institutional representative
■ Valid passport including photo identification, date of birth, and accurate spelling of the holder's name

---

Upon submission of the above, it is quite appropriate to ask for an estimate as to when the Social Security card should be received. If it does not arrive by that time, assistance can be obtained from the program administrator or from staff at the Exchange Visitor Service of ECFMG. Note that this assistance is available not only to ECFMG-sponsored J-1 visa holders but to IMGs on H-1B visas as well.

When the card is received it should be presented to the program administrator but should be retained in a safe place by the cardholder. For security reasons, an individual's SSN should not be disclosed to anyone other than those having legitimate need for it, and then only the number should be reported. The card itself need rarely be displayed.

Once an IMG has a valid SSN, the process of obtaining bank accounts, credit cards, and a driver's license is considerably easier, so this should be one of the first orders of business on arrival in the United States, but, again, not until at least 10 days after arrival.

Driver's License

A valid driver's license is legally required to operate any motor vehicle, including motorcycles and scooters; driving without one can result in a significant fine. Licenses are issued by each state, usually by the state's Department of Motor Vehicles (DMV) or an equivalent agency. Each state agency has a Web site that provides detailed information on how to obtain a license and what kinds of documents are necessary at the time of application; this is your best source of specific information. Generally, a valid passport and visa including a current I-94 form will be required along with one or more other pieces of identification and/or proof of residence within the state (e.g., utility bills, official correspondence addressed to the applicant by name at the local address). A Social Security card is not always technically required but having one often makes the application process easier.

An international driver's license obtained in the home country can be used for a limited period of time in the United States, but once residency is established in the state, there is a requirement for a license from that state. Almost all states will require the applicant to pass a written examination regarding traffic regulations and safety issues. Information to prepare for these is also available on Web sites or at the DMV offices. These are usually fairly brief multiple choice examinations, but preparation is necessary. There will also be an eye examination, so if glasses are used for driving they should be worn for the exam and must then always be worn when driving.

In some states the applicant will initially be issued a learner's permit and can only drive with an adult licensed driver in the car. Alternatively, some states will allow the applicant who has a driver's license from their home country and who has passed the written and eye exams to proceed directly to a road test. An examiner will ride with the applicant directing him or her over a standard course that usually includes parallel parking and making a three point or "broken U-turn." On successful completion, a driver's license will be issued that contains a photograph taken at that time. Most states issue licenses for several years, but in some states they will only be issued for the duration of the visa or I-94. This will most often affect J-1 visa holders, who should be prepared to apply for a renewal before their current license expires.

Getting Settled

BANK ACCOUNTS AND CREDIT CARDS

Bank Accounts

It is not advisable to carry large sums of money on one's person. Checks or cash should be deposited in a suitable commercial bank. To open a bank account, several forms of identification are needed. Most banks typically accept two or more of the items listed in Box 10-2 as proof of identification.

☑ **BOX 10-2   Proof of Identification Required for Opening Bank Account***

1. Valid passport
2. International driver's license
3. Employee photo identification card (you will receive this at orientation)
4. Employment authorization document
5. Signed copy of residency contract
6. Letter from program coordinator confirming position as a resident

*Most banks typically require at least two of these.

Consider opening both a savings and checking account and requesting a bank debit card. Debit cards allow you access to your money in checking or saving accounts so you can make purchases at shops and restaurants or withdraw money from an automatic teller machine (ATM). Many debit cards come with a credit card logo, but they are not credit cards and do not help establish credit.

Finding a suitable bank with multiple branch locations is quite easy in most cities. When selecting a bank, consider its convenience to either your training program or your residence. The same is true for automated teller machines. Make sure that the bank's ATMs are conveniently located in areas or places you will frequent if you plan to use them to make cash withdrawals or deposits.

Another safety measure and convenience is direct deposit. Most institutions or hospitals offer their employees direct deposit for their paychecks. The institution or hospital electronically directly deposits paychecks on payday to either your savings and/or checking accounts, thus eliminating the need to carry large sums of money or wait to have the check cashed. To use your bank's on-line or electronic banking features, you will need your SSN. This can easily be established at a later date.

Credit Cards

A credit card is a form of borrowing that often involves fees and specified conditions that you must understand and abide by. It is difficult to obtain a credit card if you do not have a credit history in the United States.

One of the fastest (but not necessarily the best) ways to get credit is to apply for a *secured* credit card. This requires depositing money into a savings account or certificate of deposit (CD), equivalent to the credit limit on the card, which is frozen while the card is in use. These cards often come with extra fees, so be sure to ask for all the details. Paying the monthly credit card bill on time and in full can help to establish a credit history.

An *unsecured* credit card is a pre-approved loan with interest rates. This card is issued when there is a good credit history and a demonstrated ability to repay the amount borrowed on time. The three basic types of credit cards are found in Box 10-3.

☑ BOX 10-3   Three Basic Types of Credit Cards

1. Bank cards issued by banks (e.g., Visa, MasterCard, Discover)
2. Travel and entertainment (T&E) cards (e.g., American Express, Diners Club)
3. House cards; these are valid only in one chain of stores or a single store (e.g., gas cards, local department stores)

Apply first to your own bank for a credit card because they already know you. House cards are another good place to start to begin establishing a credit history. You may find that they are more likely to offer you credit based on your salary and employment history. The fees on these cards are frequently high.

Affinity cards are bank cards that carry an organization's logo in addition to the lender's emblem. Many professional medical organizations offer these cards to its members. Ask your program coordinator if you have been enrolled as a resident member of any professional organizations, then contact that organization to see if you are eligible for an unsecured credit card. Membership fees for resident members are usually minimal and frequently less than $100/year.

Credit unions are financial institutions established by an institution or company to provide banking services to its members and may exist at larger hospitals or universities. They often offer lower fees on loans and many offer credit cards. If your institution has a credit union, you should consider using it for your banking, loans (auto or personal), and credit card needs.

If you already have a credit card issued from a large international bank, you should ask a U.S. branch of that bank about converting this into a card that can be used without the high international fees.

When establishing a credit history, the factors listed in Box 10-4 are frequently taken into consideration by many companies.

☑ **BOX 10-4   Factors in Establishing a Credit History**

1. Employment status
2. Residence history
3. Timely payments on bills and loans
4. Longevity of accounts
5. Low or no outstanding debt

When applying for a credit card, be sure to read and understand all the terms, conditions, and fees associated with the card. It is wise to search for the best possible deal. If at all possible, it is best to pay the full amount of each monthly credit card bill or as much as possible rather than the minimum required payment. Amounts not paid are subject to extremely high interest, and credit card debt can rapidly accumulate and become very difficult to pay off.

FOOD

For residents to function at their best, it is important that they eat well and sensibly. The demands of training often lead to a diet of "fast foods," which are usually not nutritionally good. Most hospitals have dining areas. In some there is a separate dining area for hospital staff, while in others there is a common dining area shared with patients and visitors. At some institutions residents receive meals as part of their contract, whereas at others residents must pay for food at the hospital. Residents also have the option of bringing food from home, which may be more economical.

Outside the hospital, residents without spouses or families may opt to take their meals in restaurants or purchase "take out" food to consume at home. However, this can be expensive, and even residents on their own should probably consider preparing at least some of their own meals. Residents with spouses and/or families will likely be eating meals prepared at home by themselves or their spouses.

In most American cities and towns, there are many options for grocery shopping. Many hospitals offer membership in large buying clubs where food and other household goods can be purchased more cheaply in bulk. However, this may not be ideal for residents on their own or with only a spouse. Large supermarkets are generally available, and many are open 24 hours a day. Shoppers who frequent a particular supermarket can obtain a free discount card for use in that supermarket. Most supermarkets have a large variety of foods, including meats, fish, and fresh fruit and vegetables. They also frequently offer at least some ethnic foods. In some areas there are farmers' markets, which often offer the freshest produce at the best prices. In addition, there are many ethnic specialty shops that offer foods from a variety of countries and cultures. Their location can be found by asking fellow residents of one's own ethnicity.

Foodstuffs are also available at smaller convenience stores and even in many gasoline stations. However, these tend to be overpriced, and shopping for food in these places is probably best done only in small quantities and only when necessary. Drugstores or pharmacies are also abundant and, in addition to prescription and nonprescription drugs, carry a wide variety of toiletries and personal-care products; many carry basic food items as well.

TRANSPORTATION

The United States is a nation of drivers and almost everyone owns and drives a car. However, it is a serious offense to drive without a valid driver's license (see above). Most people purchase cars, although it is also possible to lease a vehicle for several years. Because there are so many cars, there is a large market of available used cars—many, but certainly not all, in good condition. New cars can be purchased through an authorized car dealership. These dealerships also offer used cars, and there are some dealers who specialize in only used cars. In addition, individuals frequently advertise cars for sale in local newspapers or on bulletin boards in shops.

Buying a car, especially a used car, requires the necessary scrutiny to ensure that the vehicle is in good working order, is safe, and can be expected to function well for some time. People buying cars will frequently ask a mechanic or at least a friend with some mechanical expertise to look over the car and test drive it before they purchase. New cars and some used cars come with warranties that will cover certain types of repairs, but sometimes the warranty requires periodic maintenance of the car (which is actually an inherently good idea). Cars must also be insured and registered by their owners, usually annually. Drivers must have evidence of current insurance with them while driving the car, and the car must display valid license plates and registration stickers. At the time of or before registration, they must also undergo safety and emission inspections, and certificates of successful inspection are required. All of these require payment of fees.

Americans are often known for the size of their cars and certainly there is a selection of sport-utility vehicles, station wagons, and minivans, but there are also smaller and more economical options. The number of people expected to be riding in the car, the cost of the car, the planned frequency of use of the car, and its condition should all be factored into the decision of which car to purchase.

Newly arriving IMGs should also be aware that driving under the influence of alcohol (DUI) is a very serious offense and can result in arrest and loss of the driving license. It could also jeopardize one's medical license. In addition, almost all states require that occupants wear seatbelts while driving and that children be put in properly designed child restraints in the rear seat. In the event that a driver is pulled over by the police, it is imperative to remain in the car with both hands on the steering wheel and to await the officer's questions and directions. Other actions can be misinterpreted as threatening and could lead to a potentially dangerous reaction by the officer.

Public transportation is more variable; it is quite well developed in larger urban areas but often nonexistent in suburban or rural areas. Buses and commuter trains generally operate on fixed schedules with regular, clearly identified stops for passengers to board and disembark. Often it is possible to purchase a card that allows a rider to dispense with paying a fare on each trip. Otherwise, fares are typically paid on boarding the bus or train or entering a station and often require exact change.

Other options for transportation include motorcycles and scooters for the more daring and bicycles when the weather and distance permit. The latter is also an excellent way to stay in good physical condition.

Rush hours, at the beginning and end of the typical workday, can result in delays for both drivers and riders of public transportation, and sufficient time should always be left to arrive at the hospital on time for morning rounds and conferences. Additional travel time should be allowed during inclement weather.

PERSONAL HEALTH CARE

While the residents are primarily focused on the health of their patients, they must also pay attention to their own health needs as well as those of their spouses and/or dependents. By ACGME requirement, all GME programs must provide health and dental insurance for residents and their dependents; this insurance is usually adequate. Program administrators can provide information on health care plans, including what services are covered and any options for additional care. Fees for this coverage are usually deducted directly from the resident's paycheck.

Residents are also permitted a number of "sick days" each year. These should only be taken when the resident is actually unable to function or may be in a contagious state. In such instances, residents must call in to their supervisors as soon as they realize they will be unable to work and give a realistic projection as to when they will return to work. Using sick days for minor illnesses or other inappropriate reasons puts a strain on those who must cover for the absent resident, will engender ill feelings, and could lead to disciplinary action.

RELIGIOUS ACTIVITIES

The United States has a very proud tradition of religious freedom, which was one of the main incentives to originally establish this country. There is also a separation of church and state, which means that there is no official state religion and all religions may be freely practiced.

The range of churches, temples, mosques, and other houses of worship available in any given area is variable but is most related to the size and diversity of the community. Religious institutions can be found by consulting local telephone directories or simply by asking people at the hospital or in one's neighborhood where a particular denomination may be located.

American churches, temples, and mosques often serve as a focal point for the community. Many have schools associated with them as well as social activities for their members and friends. They are also often places to meet people from one's home country or culture.

All people in America are entitled to practice their religion freely. If there are religious restrictions on diet, working during certain time periods, participating in certain medical procedures, or other requirements such as praying periodically, they must be respected in the workplace and reasonable accommodations made for the individual. However, if these result in a resident not being able to perform certain activities or work at certain times, this information should be provided to the program director well in advance of the situation arising.

Recreational Activities

There is an old adage that says, "All work and no play makes Jack a dull boy." Thus, despite the demands of a rigorous training program, it is essential that IMGs make time and effort to engage in recreational activities outside of medicine. This will help them to maintain their own mental health and, as they come to learn and understand American culture through these activities, they will find it easier to relate and converse with both medical colleagues and patients.

INDIVIDUAL ACTIVITIES

The range of recreational activities and diversions available to any resident is almost limitless. For the individual, physical fitness can often be a challenge when working long hours with limited days off. Hence, it is wise to combine fitness and recreation into some enjoyable activities that will also enhance conditioning. Almost any imaginable sport or physical activity can be pursued, limited only by time, energy, and in some cases, weather.

Cycling is an excellent way to get some exercise and see the local areas up close, and can even serve as a means of transportation. Jogging or running is very popular and requires no special equipment or expertise. 5K and 10K fun races are frequently held and a good way to meet people. Tennis and golf are also popular among physicians but require a bit more time and talent.

Many hospitals provide fitness facilities with aerobic exercise machines and weights, or one can join a local fitness facility. Similarly, classes like yoga may be available.

The number of movies and television shows available is overwhelming. And, whether by watching television or attending in person, Americans are avid sports spectators. Baseball, once inarguably the "national pastime", now battles with football, basketball, and hockey for fans' attention. Fortunately, the four major sports have different, although slightly overlapping, seasons. The Super Bowl, the professional football championship game, is a sporting and social event of epic proportions. Americans tend to be very loyal, sometimes almost rabid, fans of their home teams. IMG residents who can learn even a little about the players and recent performances of the local teams will find a very effective way of establishing some personal connection with American colleagues and patients alike. However, they should not expect Americans to be knowledgeable about what they call soccer (what the rest of the world calls football) or cricket!

GROUP ACTIVITIES AND MEETING PEOPLE

Coming to a new country can be a lonely experience for an IMG and possibly even more so for his or her spouse. Most programs make an attempt to welcome newcomers. Often there will be social gatherings at the beginning of the program and periodically through the year where residents can come together with their spouses and families to relax and enjoy themselves.

In some instances there will be social organizations based around ethnicities or cultures where people from one's home country can be found and familiar food, drink, and music can be enjoyed. However, restricting social activity only to one's own ethnic group can be limiting: IMGs should make efforts to get out and meet Americans and people of other ethnicities. As mentioned above, religious institutions also provide the opportunity to meet different kinds of people. Additionally, IMGs who have children in school will find it much easier to develop social contacts by meeting other parents.

Possibly the biggest social challenge is that which faces the IMG who arrives with no spouse or family and is in a program with few other IMGs or few from his or her own country or culture. All of the above activities are possible ways of making friends. Most urban areas also have a large number of dance and music clubs where young adults from all walks of life come together to enjoy each other's company. Dating and simple activities like dinner and a movie are common ways for people to get to know each other. Although it is not inappropriate to date people from one's program or hospital, it is important to maintain professional relations at all times in the workplace. Unwanted advances may be considered a form of sexual harassment. Information and guidelines regarding this topic are generally included in initial orientation for all new hospital staff. Strict sanctions do, however, exist against doctors dating patients.

TRAVEL

The United States is a vast country with diverse geography and climates. Regardless of visa status, there is no impediment to traveling freely from state to state. The bigger constraint is obviously time and money.

Using one's vacation time to travel throughout the United States is an excellent way to see many of its natural wonders and to meet its people. National and state parks are popular tourist sites. Major cities like New York, Chicago, Washington, and San Francisco are certainly worth seeing and experiencing. America has an abundance of beaches and lakes for warm weather activity as well as snowy resorts for winter activities. For those with children, a visit to Disneyland in California or Walt Disney World in Florida is almost inevitable.

There are many travel agencies both locally and online that can assist in planning itineraries and booking accommodations. Perhaps the biggest pitfall is to attempt to do and see too much and to arrive back to work exhausted instead of relaxed. Sometimes it is more restful to plan short weekend getaways to areas closer to home. Co-workers may be the best source of information regarding such trips.

Although visa status is not an issue with respect to travel within America, it is an issue with respect to international travel, particularly with respect to re-entry into the United States. Specific information on international travel while on a visa can be found in Chapter 4.

Family Considerations

For the IMG who is coming to the United States to enter GME training and who has a spouse, children, and/or an extended family, there are some difficult decisions to be made.

SHOULD SPOUSE/FAMILY ACCOMPANY THE IMG?

The first decision is whether or not the spouse and/or family will accompany the IMG in his or her emigration to the United States. Residencies are at least three years in duration, and many are much longer; travel back to the home country during that training period may be restricted by time, cost, and visa issues. Hence, leaving spouse and children behind means that there will be long periods with no contact over several years.

SPOUSE EMPLOYMENT/EDUCATIONAL OPTIONS

Dependents of IMGs with J-1 visa status typically have J-2 visa status and may seek employment in the United States. However, they must first file an Application for Employment Authorization (Form I-765) with Citizenship and Immigration Services. Permission for employment will be granted only provided that the earned income is not needed for support of the principle (J-1) Exchange Visitor. Form I-765 may be obtained by accessing the USCIS home page at www.uscis.gov. In contrast, neither the spouse nor the dependents of IMGs on H-1B visas are permitted to work.

There are no restrictions on spouses pursuing educational opportunities at any level, although some state universities may have residency requirements. There are also a large number of community colleges and private institutions where spouses may enroll, although tuition at private colleges and universities can be quite high. Many will offer financial assistance to qualifying individuals.

SCHOOLS

IMGs who are accompanied by school-age children must make provision for enrolling them in appropriate schools. The United States has a very extensive system of public and private schools. Public schools are tuition-free, but attendance at a particular school/school district is determined by the location of the child's residence. In so far as the quality of education can vary considerably even in the adjacent districts, this may often be a factor in the decision about where to rent or buy an apartment or home. This information is best obtained from individuals in the program who have children enrolled in local schools.

Private schools generally do not place any restriction on the child's place of residence but may not always be able to accommodate the child. Tuition at private schools can also be quite high. Subsets of private schools are those operated by a religious denomination or sect. Although children attending such schools do not necessarily have to come from families of that same denomination or sect, parents should be aware that they will likely receive religious instruction as part of the curriculum.

Elementary schools typically offer classes beginning at the kindergarten level. Middle schools usually encompass grades six through eight, high schools grades nine through twelve. The specific design of a school system is a function of the local school district and can vary considerably from district to district.

It is also common practice to enroll younger children in preschool classes. This may begin at any age, and preschoolers may attend anywhere from a few hours to a full day up to five days per week. As important as the preschool experience is for children, it may be even more important when both parents are employed outside the home or the child is being raised by a single parent, both of which scenarios are common in American society.

Although having children enrolled in local schools can be challenging, it also presents an excellent opportunity for parents to meet other parents and become integrated into the local community. Parents should also be aware that most schools have extensive after-school and weekend events and programs, including sports activities. This can lead to a great deal of time and effort shuttling and collecting children from these activities, sometimes referred to as the "soccer mom (or dad)" syndrome.

Emergency Assistance

Throughout the United States, there is a dedicated telephone number, **911**, that can be used to summon emergency assistance from police or fire departments or to contact emergency medical care providers. This number can be dialed for free from any telephone anywhere in the United States and provides immediate contact. If you need to use it, remain calm and tell the operator the nature of your emergency and where you are. Stay on the line and follow any instructions. *Do not use this number for anything other than true emergencies.*

Getting Local Information

Many of the issues addressed in this chapter vary considerably depending on the location and nature of the program that the IMG is entering. Often, the best source of information is IMGs already in that program or at least in the local area. Unfortunately, the opportunity to pose practical questions and receive advice does not occur until the IMG arrives in the United States, only weeks or days before starting the program. Relatives and colleagues who have preceded the IMG and who are acclimatized to the American way of life may be helpful. Depending on their visa status, some IMGs may qualify to participate in the ECFMG IMG Advisors Network (IAN) (www.ecfmg.org/acculturation) and be put in direct contact with IMGs in the United States months before they need to leave their home country. Some ethnic medical societies also provide advisors and mentors for IMGs coming from their countries or geographical areas. Contact information for the ECFMG program and ethnic medical societies can be found in Appendix D.

Appendix A

Glossary of Frequently Used Terms, Abbreviations, and Acronyms

Medical, Professional, and Educational Organizations

AAFP	American Academy of Family Physicians
AAMC	Association of American Medical Colleges
AAP	American Academy of Pediatrics
ABFM	American Board of Family Medicine
ABIM	American Board of Internal Medicine
ABMS	American Board of Medical Specialties
ABP	American Board of Pediatrics
ACGME	Accreditation Council for Graduate Medical Education
ACP	American College of Physicians
ACS	American College of Surgeons
AHA	American Hospital Association
AMA	American Medical Association
AOA	American Osteopathic Association
FSMB	Federation of State Medical Boards
IOM	Institute of Medicine
NIH	National Institute of Health
RRC	Residency Review Committee

Examination, Certification, and Application Organizations and Terms

CAF	Common Application Form (used in ERAS)
CAQ	Certificate of Added Qualifications
CK	Clinical Knowledge (USMLE Step 2 CK examination)
CS	Clinical Skills (USMLE Step 2 CS Examination)
CSEC	Clinical Skills Evaluation Collaboration
CVS	Certification Verification Service
ECFMG	Educational Commission for Foreign Medical Graduates
ERAS	Electronic Residency Application System
IMED	International Medical Education Directory
IWA	Interactive Web Application
LOR	Letter of Recommendation
MSPE	Medical Student Performance Evaluation (replaced Dean's Letter)
NBME	National Board of Medical Examiners
NRMP	National Residency Matching Program (commonly referred to as "The Match")
OASIS	Online Application Status and Information System
ROL	Rank Order List
Scramble	The period when NRMP applicants who do not match can contact and apply to programs with unmatched positions (see ERAS)

SP	Standardized Patient
Specialty Board Examinations	Examinations administered by ABMS Specialty Boards used in determination of whether a resident successfully completing specialty training will be certified as a specialist in a Specialty or Subspecialty (often referred to simply as "The Boards"). Depending on specialty, there may be one or more examinations.
TOEFL	Test of English as a Foreign Language
TSE	Test of Spoken English
USMLE	United States Medical Licensing Examination

Immigration Terms

EVSP	Exchange Visitor Sponsorship Program
Green Card	Lawful Permanent Resident
H-1B	Non-Immigrant Work Visa or Temporary Worker in Specialized Occupation
HPSA	Health Professions Shortage Areas
J-1 Visa	Exchange Visitor Visa

Program and Institutional Terms

ACLS	Advanced Cardiac Life Support (AHA program)
ATLS	Advanced Trauma Life Support (ACS program)
Attending	Fully licensed and certified physician, usually with faculty appointment, who has ultimate responsibility for patient care and teaching on a medical or surgical service
Call/On-call	Assigned hours when a resident or fellow is either on duty in a hospital or available to come to the hospital
Categorical	GME program in which it is anticipated that the resident will complete the full course of training, assuming satisfactory performance
Chief Resident	The most senior resident(s) in a GME program, often spending an additional year and assuming increased administrative and teaching responsibilities
Clerkship	*See* Externship
Consultant	Physician specialist called in to consult on a particular patient
DME	Director of Medical Education
EMT	Emergency Medical Technician
ER/ED	Emergency Room/Emergency Department
Externship	A clinical experience for U.S. or international medical students or international medical graduates in which they participate in supervised patient care in a clinical department for a period of time, usually one month (*see also* Clerkship, Subinternship)
Fellow	Physician pursuing training in a medical subspecialty, usually after completion of a residency in a relevant specialty
GME	Graduate Medical Education
Housestaff	A term used for physicians-in-training at all levels (but not medical students)
IMG	International Medical Graduate
In-Training Examination	Specialty examinations administered by ABMS Specialty Boards or Specialty Societies to assist residents and PDs in assessing resident and program standings relative to national standards
Intern	First Postgraduate Year (an older term, less commonly used now)
IRB	Institutional Review Board
Joint Commission	Formerly, the Joint Commission on Accreditation of Healthcare Organizations
LVN/LPN	Licensed Vocational Nurse/Licensed Practical Nurse

MSW	Medical Social Worker
Observership	A clinical experience for international medical students or international medical graduates in which they observe, but cannot participate in, patient care in a clinical department
OR	Operating Room
OSHA	Occupational Safety and Health Administration
OT	Occupational Therapist
Paramedic	Pre-hospital care provider with advanced skills and training
PD	Program Director
PGY	Postgraduate Year (e.g., PGY-1 = first year, PGY-2 = second year; sometimes shortened to PG1, PG2, etc.)
Preliminary	A GME program providing only one year of training; subsequently a resident must obtain or have another position in another GME program
Primary Care Physician	A health care provider who acts as a first point of consultation for all patients.
PT	Physical Therapist
QI	Quality Improvement
Resident	Physician participating in an initial graduate medical education program
RN	Registered Nurse
Rotation	A defined period of time (usually one month or four weeks) during which a resident is assigned to a particular service or area of the hospital
Specialty	A medical or surgical area of concentration (e.g., Internal Medicine, General Surgery, Pediatrics)
Subinternship	See Externship
Subspecialty	A more limited and specialized area of concentration within a medical or surgical specialty (e.g., Cardiology, Pediatric Surgery)
TPL	Training Program Liaison (liaison between J-1 residents and ECFMG)
Unit	An area of a hospital providing specialized and advanced care (e.g., Medical Intensive Care Unit [MICU], Coronary Care Unit [CCU], Pediatric Intensive Care Unit [PICU])

Appendix B

Internet Web Sites

Listed below are Web site addresses (URLs) for organizations and sites that may provide useful information relevant to the material in the chapters under which they are listed. Within the chapters are more specific URLs, but the same material can be reached by searching the Web sites below. In addition, most material can be found by using standard search engines such as www.google.com.

Chapter 1

Accreditation Council for Graduate Medical Education
www.acgme.org

Osteopathic Physicians
www.do-online.org

Chapter 2

Educational Commission for Foreign Medical Graduates (ECFMG)
www.ecfmg.org

Foundation for Advancement of International Medical Education (FAIMER)
(contains International Medical Education Directory [IMED])
www.faimer.org

U.S. Medical Licensing Examination
www.usmle.org

Educational Testing Service
www.ets.org

National Board of Medical Examiners
www.nbme.org

American College of Physicians
www.acponline.org

Federation of State Medical Boards
www.fsmb.org

American Medical Association
www.ama-assn.org

Chapter 3

Graduate Management Admission Council (GMAC)
www.mba.com/mba

Association of American Medical Colleges
www.aamc.org (search MSPE guide)

American Academy of Family Practice
www.aafp.org (search Letters of Reference)

Electronic Residency Application Service
www.aamc.org/eras

ERAS Support at ECFMG
www.ecfmg.org/eras
eras-support@ecfmg.org (e-mail)

National Resident Matching Program
www.nrmp.org

San Francisco Match
www.sfmatch.org

Chapter 4

Department of State (search Visas, Waivers)
http://travel.state.gov

Embassies, Consulates, and Diplomatic Missions
usembassy.state.gov.

Exchange Visitor Program
http://exchanges.state.gov/education/jexchanges/

ECFMG Exchange Visitor Program
www.ecfmg.org/evsp

Citizenship and Immigration Services
www.uscis.gov

Department of Homeland Security
www.dhs.gov/dhspublic

Chapter 5

Virtual Mentor (AMA)
www.virtualmentor.org

Calgary – Cambridge Guide to the Medical Interview – Communication Process
www.gp-training.net/training/theory/calgary/calgary.pdf

Educational Testing Service
www.ets.org

English for International Opportunity
www.ielts.org

Patient-Centered Communication
www.ama-assn.org/ama/pub/category/11929.html

Chapter 6

ECFMG Acculturation Program
www.ecfmg.org/acculturation

Chapter 7

American College of Physicians – Health Tips
foundation.acponline.org/hl/htips.htm

Accreditation Council for Graduate Medical Education (ACGME)
www.acgme.org

Institute for Healthcare Improvement (IHI)
www.ihi.org

Chapter 8

National Library of Medicine
www.nlm.nih.gov

PubMed
www.ncbi.nlm.nih.gov/PubMed/

The Cochrane Collaboration
www.cochrane.org

EMBase
www.embase.com

Agency for Healthcare Research and Quality
www.ahrq.gov/

American Academy of Family Practice
www.aafp.org/online/en/home/residents.html

American Academy of Pediatrics
www.aap.org/sections/ypn/r/

American Board of Medical Specialties (ABMS)
www.abms.org

Plagiarism
www.plagiarism.org
www.tunitin.com

Research Integrity
ori.dhhs.gov/
www.cgsnet.org

Centers for Medicare and Medicaid Services
www.cms.hhs.gov

Department of Veterans Affairs
www.va.gov

Chapter 9

American Board of Internal Medicine
www.abim.org

Federation of State Medical Boards
www.fsmb.org

National Practitioner Data Bank
www.npdb-hipdb.com

Centers for Medicare and Medicaid Services
www.cms.hhs.gov

Drug Enforcement Administration – Diversion Control
www.deadiversion.usdoj.gov

Internal Revenue Service
www.irs.gov

American Board of Medical Specialties (ABMS)
www.abms.org

Chapter 10

Social Security Administration
www.socialsecurity.gov

Citizen and Immigration Services
www.uscis.gov

ECFMG Acculturation Program
www.ecfmg.org/acculturation

References

American Medical Association. **Graduate Medical Education Directory, including programs accredited by the Accreditation Council for Graduate Medical Education.** AMA Press: Chicago; 2006.

Association of American Medical Colleges. **Roadmap to Residency: From Application to the Match and Beyond, 2nd ed [PDF].** AAMC: Washington, DC; 2007.

Bigby JA, ed. **Cross-Cultural Medicine.** Philadelphia: American College of Physicians; 2003.

Chander K. **First Aid for the International Medical Graduate.** McGraw-Hill: New York; 2002.

Iserson KV. **Iserson's Getting into a Residency: A Guide from Medical Students, 7th ed.** Galen Press: Tucson, AZ; 2000.

Lanier AR. **Living in the USA, 6th ed.** Revised by JC Davis. Intercultural Press: Yarmouth, MA; 2005.

Livingston M. **Newcomer's Handbook for Moving to and Living in the USA.** First Books: Portland, OR; 2005.

Purnell LD, Paulanka BJ. **Transcultural Health Care: A Culturally Competent Approach, 2nd ed.** FA Davis: Philadelphia; 2003.

Storti C. **Cross-Cultural Dialogues: 74 Brief Encounters with Cultural Differences.** Intercultural Press: Yarmouth, MA; 1994.

Verghese A. **My Own Country: A Doctor's Story.** Random House: New York; 1995.

Appendix D

Educational Commission for Foreign Medical Graduates (ECFMG) Resources

ECFMG Certification
- Visit the ECFMG Web site at www.ecfmg.org for access to important updates, the Interactive Web Application (IWA), and publications, including:
  - ECFMG *Information Booklet*
  - ECFMG *Certification Fact Sheet*
  - *International Medical Education Directory* (IMED)
  - *The ECFMG Reporter*
- Visit the USMLE Web site at www.usmle.org for its *Bulletin of Information*, important updates, and sample test and orientation materials.
- Visit the NBME Web site at www.nbme.org for USMLE self-assessment services.

Electronic Residency Application Service (ERAS) Support Services at ECFMG
- Web site: www.ecfmg.org/eras
- E-mail: eras-support@ecfmg.org
- Telephone: (215) 386-5900
  (*Telephone assistance is available between 9:00 A.M. and 5:00 P.M. Eastern Time, Monday through Friday.*)

Exchange Visitor Sponsorship Program (EVSP)
- Web site: www.ecfmg.org/evsp
- ECFMG *J-1 Visa Sponsorship Fact Sheet*, available on the website.
- Telephone: (215) 823-2121
  (*Telephone assistance is available between 9:00 A.M. and 5:00 P.M. Eastern Time, Monday through Friday.*)

ECFMG Acculturation Program
- Web site: www.ecfmg.org/acculturation
- E-mail: acculturation@ecfmg.org

General Information and Inquiries
- Web site: www.ecfmg.org
- E-mail: info@ecfmg.org
- Telephone: (215) 386-5900
  (*Telephone assistance is available between 9:00 A.M. and 5:00 P.M. Eastern Time, Monday through Friday.*)
- Mailing address:
  Educational Commission for Foreign Medical Graduates
  3624 Market Street
  Philadelphia, PA 19104-2685
  USA

The ECFMG IMG Advisors Network (IAN)

The Educational Commission for Foreign Medical Graduates (ECFMG) has begun a series of initiatives designed to facilitate the transition of international medical graduates (IMGs) arriving from outside the United States into U.S. medicine and culture. These efforts are in response to the growing recognition that, even though many IMGs arrive with excellent prior medical education and fluency in English, there are still many issues that are confusing and unclear. The U.S. health care system and the institutions where IMGs train may be organized and operate very differently from those with which they are familiar. They must learn to live and work in the United States and adjust to differences in language and culture. This transition can be quite stressful not only for the physician but for family members accompanying the IMG.

   Most IMGs do make the necessary transitions and eventually become comfortable working in hospitals and clinics and living in the United States. However, ECFMG's discussions with focus groups of IMGs indicate that this transition could be facilitated by

- Advice from other IMGs who have entered U.S. training programs, who can provide practical and useful answers to questions and concerns on a wide range of topics.
- Access to this advice and other acculturation resources before leaving the home country, where these resources may be limited, and before the demands and challenges of the new training program begin.

To accomplish this, ECFMG has established the IMG Advisors Network.

IMG Advisors Network

The IMG Advisors Network (IAN) is a free service that allows qualified IMGs who will be coming to the United States from other countries to connect with advisors who can answer questions about living and working in the United States. To use this service to obtain advice, you must meet the qualifications of advisees. There are also qualifications for advisors, which include being in or having completed an ACGME-accredited training program in the United States.

   IAN advisors serve on a volunteer basis. The IAN database lists available advisors by name, medical specialty, U.S. GME institution, location in the United States, country of medical education, medical school, and other demographics. IMGs using this service can select one or more advisors based on these criteria. Once advisors have been selected, the e-mail address of the IMG seeking advice will be provided to the advisors, who can then begin communicating directly with the advisee.

   The communications between advisors and advisees are direct, rather than through ECFMG. However, there is an option to copy ECFMG on any particular e-mail, if the advisor or advisee chooses to do so. The purpose for this is simply to allow IAN staff to see what kinds of issues are being raised and to use that information to develop more and better resources to assist IMGs throughout the acculturation process. There will be no response from ECFMG to such "cc's". If you choose not to copy ECFMG, correspondence between advisor and advisee will not be visible to or monitored by ECFMG.

Nature of Advice

There is a wide range of topics that might be raised by advisees and could be addressed appropriately by advisors. A sample of such topics includes

- Bringing spouses or family right away versus having them come after getting settled
- When to arrive
- Where to find lodging
- Where to find ethnic restaurants and grocery stores
- Where to find houses of worship
- Setting up personal finances (e.g., bank accounts, credit cards, Social Security Numbers)
- Advisability of getting a driver's license and buying an automobile
- What to pack (e.g., kinds and amount of clothes, personal effects)
- Spouse and children concerns (e.g., employment opportunities, child care, schools)
- Support groups (i.e., people from the same country or ethnic group)
- What to expect as far as work and call schedules, time off, vacations
- Recreational resources
- American culture (e.g., books, TV shows, movies, music, sports)
- Language (e.g., idioms, jargon, abbreviations; ECFMG will be developing and making available materials in these areas)
- Unique features or characteristics of the program or the area in which it is located

Some topics should *not* be discussed with advisors:

- Questions regarding the ECFMG Certification process. The policies and procedures related to ECFMG Certification are complex and subject to change. For these inquiries, advisees should refer to the ECFMG Web site or contact ECFMG's Applicant Information Services at info@ecfmg.org or (215) 386-5900.
- Questions regarding participation in or application to ECFMG's J-1 Exchange Visitor Sponsorship Program. The requirements for ECFMG J-1 visa sponsorship and the related federal regulations are complex. Advisees should refer these issues to ECFMG's Exchange Visitor Sponsorship department at (215) 823-2121 or visit www.ecfmg.org/evsp/index.html. Discussion and advice regarding the various visa options for physicians may be an area in which the advisors might contribute; however, ECFMG discourages IAN advisors from providing specific immigration counseling.
- Although advisors can provide advice regarding preparation for the USMLE examinations, including USMLE Step 3, they must never disclose actual test material, such as questions, test cases, or other specific test content. IMGs receiving such information would be at risk of sanction for irregular behavior and could have their records permanently annotated or be subject to bars from future examinations.
- Advisors will defer to program directors or program administrators if advice or information differs from that the IMG might receive directly from the program director or program or institution staff.

Participation in IAN is limited to those IMGs who have applied to ECFMG for initial J-1 visa sponsorship. To participate in IAN, advisees must

- Be certified by ECFMG,
- Have been offered a position in an ACGME-accredited training program, and

- Have submitted an application and payment to the ECFMG Exchange Visitor Sponsorship Program for initial sponsorship as a J-1 Alien Physician.

IMGs eligible to participate in IAN as an advisee should receive an e-mail directly from the ECFMG Exchange Visitor Sponsorship Program indicating receipt of their J-1 application and fee and directing them to www.ecfmg.org/acculturation for more information and directions for enrolling and selecting advisors.

The program also accepts new advisors on an ongoing basis. IAN advisers must

- Be certified by ECFMG
- Either be enrolled in or have completed training in an ACGME-accredited program
- Be licensed to practice medicine (training or permanent license) in at least one state or jurisdiction in the United States
- Have ready access to e-mail
- Be willing to reply to inquiries from advisees in an honest and timely manner

Interested potential IAN advisors should go to the aforementioned Web site (www.ecfmg.org/acculturation) for more information and directions on how to participate.

Ethnic Medical Societies

National Arab American Medical Association
801 S. Adams Street, Suite 208
Birmingham, MI 48009
(248) 646-3661
www.naama.com

National Hispanic Medical Association
1700 17th Street NW, Suite 405
Washington, DC 20009
(202) 265-4297
www.nhmamd.org/

North American Taiwan Medical Association - Chicago Chapter
38 Ridgefield Lane
Willowbrook, IL 60521
(708) 229-5812

Peruvian American Medical Society
4488 Tamerland Drive
West Bloomfield, MI 48322
(813) 785-5677
www.pamsnational.org

Philippine Medical Association of America
572 East 17th Street
Brooklyn, NY 11226
(718) 852-8564

Philippine Medical Association of Southern California
13352 S. Hawthorne Blvd.
Hawthorne, CA 90250
(310) 973-8863

Philippine Medical Society of Northern California
8555 San Rafael Rd.
Atascadero, CA 93422
(805) 466-4261

Polish-American Medical Society
5428 N. Milwaukee Ave.
Chicago, IL 60630
(773) 594-1515
www.zlpchicago.org

Rajasthan Medical Alumni Association
89 Shore Road
Manhasset, NY 11030
(516) 825-5505

Romanian Medical Society of New York
21-26 Broadway
Astoria, NY 11106
(718) 932-1700

Russian American Medical Assocation
36100 Euclid Avenue, Suite 330-B
Willoughby, OH 44094
(440) 953-8055
www.russiandoctors.org

Salvadorean American Medical Society
221 W. Colorado Avenue, Suite 424
Dallas, TX 75208
(305) 412-9435
www.samsdoctors.com

Semmelweis Scientific Society
863 Park Avenue
New York, NY 10028
(212) 831-3332

Serbian-American Medical Society
30 N. Michigan Avenue, Suite 510
Chicago, IL 60602
(312) 422-1033

Society of Asian-Indian Surgeons of America
Department of Surgery
Bronx Lebanon Hospital Center
Bronx, NY 10457
(718) 960-1251

Society of Philippine Surgeons in America
3629 Loggerhead Court
Seabrook Island, SC 29455
(616) 451-4240
www.spsatoday.com/index.html

Spanish-American Medical Society
420 Lakeville Road
Lake Success, NY 11042
(516) 354-0710

Thai Physicians Association of America
1165 Stonewall Trail
Fairview Heights, IL 62208
(618) 628-0223
www.tpaa.us

Turkish American Physicians Association
1350 Lexington Avenue
New York, NY 10128
(212) 697-2813

Ukrainian Medical Association of North American
2247 West Chicago Avenue
Chicago, IL 60622
(773) 278-6262
www.umana.org

United States Colombian Medical Association (USCMA)
280 Aragon Avenue
Coral Gables, FL 33134
(305) 446-7099

Venezuelan American Medical Association
P.O. Box 15460
Plantation, FL 33318-5460

Vietnamese Medical Association of the USA
4221 Greenway
Baltimore, MD
(410) 502-5382
www.vamausa.org

A Patient's Bill of Rights

American Hospital Association
Management Advisory
A Patient's Bill of Rights
Adopted by the AHA in 1973.
This revision approved by the AHA Board of Trustees on 21 October 1992.

Introduction

Effective health care requires collaboration between patients and physicians and other health care professionals. Open and honest communication, respect for personal and professional values, and sensitivity to differences are integral to optimal patient care. As the setting for the provision of health services, hospitals must provide a foundation for understanding and respecting the rights and responsibilities of patients, their families, physicians, and other caregivers. Hospitals must ensure a health care ethic that respects the role of patients in decision-making about treatment choices and other aspects of their care. Hospitals must be sensitive to cultural, racial, linguistic, religious, age, gender, and other differences as well as the needs of persons with disabilities.

The American Hospital Association presents A Patient's Bill of Rights with the expectation that it will contribute to more effective patient care and be supported by the hospital on behalf of the institution, its medical staff, employees, and patients. The American Hospital Association encourages health care institutions to tailor this bill of rights to their patient community by translating and/or simplifying the language of this bill of rights as may be necessary to ensure that patients and their families understand their rights and responsibilities.

Bill of Rights

These rights can be exercised on the patient's behalf by a designated surrogate or proxy decision maker if the patient lacks decision-making capacity, is legally incompetent, or is a minor.

1. The patient has the right to considerate and respectful care.
2. The patient has the right to and is encouraged to obtain from physicians and other direct caregivers relevant, current, and understandable information concerning diagnosis, treatment, and prognosis.

     Except in emergencies when the patient lacks decision-making capacity and the need for treatment is urgent, the patient is entitled to the opportunity to discuss and request information related to the specific procedures and/or treatments, the risks involved, the possible length of recuperation, and the medically reasonable alternatives and their accompanying risks and benefits.

     Patients have the right to know the identity of physicians, nurses, and others involved in their care, as well as when those involved are students, residents, or other trainees. The patient also has the right to know the immediate and long-term financial implications of treatment choices, insofar as they are known.

     The patient has the right to make decisions about the plan of care prior to and during the course of treatment and to refuse a recommended treatment or plan of care to the extent permitted by law and hospital policy and to be informed of the medical consequences of this action. In case of such refusal, the patient is entitled to other appropriate care and services that the hospital provides or transfer to another hospital. The hospital should notify patients of any policy that might affect patient choice within the institution.

3. The patient has the right to have an advance directive (such as a living will, health care proxy, or durable power of attorney for health care) concerning treatment or designating a surrogate decision maker with the expectation that the hospital will honor the intent of that directive to the extent permitted by law and hospital policy.

   Health care institutions must advise patients of their rights under state law and hospital policy to make informed medical choices, ask if the patient has an advance directive, and include that information in patient records. The patient has the right to timely information about hospital policy that may limit its ability to implement fully a legally valid advance directive.

   The patient has the right to every consideration of privacy. Case discussion, consultation, examination, and treatment should be conducted so as to protect each patient's privacy.

4. The patient has the right to expect that all communications and records pertaining to his/her care will be treated as confidential by the hospital, except in cases such as suspected abuse and public health hazards when reporting is permitted or required by law. The patient has the right to expect that the hospital will emphasize the confidentiality of this information when it releases it to any other parties entitled to review information in these records.

5. The patient has the right to review the records pertaining to his/her medical care and to have the information explained or interpreted as necessary, except when restricted by law.

6. The patient has the right to expect that, within its capacity and policies, a hospital will make reasonable response to the request of a patient for appropriate and medically indicated care and services. The hospital must provide evaluation, service, and/or referral as indicated by the urgency of the case. When medically appropriate and legally permissible, or when a patient has so requested, a patient may be transferred to another facility. The institution to which the patient is to be transferred must first have accepted the patient for transfer. The patient must also have the benefit of complete information and explanation concerning the need for, risks, benefits, and alternatives to such a transfer.

7. The patient has the right to ask and be informed of the existence of business relationships among the hospital, educational institutions, other health care providers, or payers that may influence the patient's treatment and care.

8. The patient has the right to consent to or decline to participate in proposed research studies or human experimentation affecting care and treatment or requiring direct patient involvement, and to have those studies fully explained prior to consent. A patient who declines to participate in research or experimentation is entitled to the most effective care that the hospital can otherwise provide.

9. The patient has the right to expect reasonable continuity of care when appropriate and to be informed by physicians and other caregivers of available and realistic patient care options when hospital care is no longer appropriate.

10. The patient has the right to be informed of hospital policies and practices that relate to patient care, treatment, and responsibilities. The patient has the right to be informed of available resources for resolving disputes, grievances, and conflicts, such as ethics committees, patient representatives, or other mechanisms available in the institution. The patient has the right to be informed of the hospital's charges for services and available payment methods.

The collaborative nature of health care requires that patients, or their families/surrogates, participate in their care. The effectiveness of care and patient satisfaction with the course of treatment depend, in part, on the patient fulfilling certain responsibilities. Patients are responsible for providing information about past illnesses, hospitalizations, medications, and other matters related to health status. To participate effectively in decision making, patients must be encouraged to take responsibility for requesting additional information or clarification about their health status or treatment when they do not fully understand information and instructions. Patients are also responsible for ensuring that the health care institution has a copy of their written advance directive if they have one. Patients are responsible for informing their physicians and other caregivers if they anticipate problems in following prescribed treatment.

Patients should also be aware of the hospital's obligation to be reasonably efficient and equitable in providing care to other patients and the community. The hospital's rules and regulations are designed to help the hospital meet this obligation. Patients and their families are responsible for making reasonable accommodations to the needs of the hospital, other patients, medical staff, and hospital employees. Patients are responsible for providing necessary information for insurance claims and for working with the hospital to make payment arrangements, when necessary.

A person's health depends on much more than health care services. Patients are responsible for recognizing the impact of their life-style on their personal health.

Conclusion

Hospitals have many functions to perform, including the enhancement of health status, health promotion, and the prevention and treatment of injury and disease; the immediate and ongoing care and rehabilitation of patients; the education of health professionals, patients, and the community; and research. All these activities must be conducted with an overriding concern for the values and dignity of patients.

Index

A

AAMC. *See* Association of American Medical Colleges
Abbreviations, 201–203
ABMS. *See* American Board of Medical Specialties
Academic dishonesty, 77
Academic integrity, 167
Account, bank, 191–192
Accreditation Council for Graduate Medical Education (ACGME), 5, 140–144
  administrative structure of, 135
  core competencies and, 141–143
  core competencies of, 29–31
  duty hours and, 143–144
  mission of education and, 92
  overview of, 140–141
  on working within team, 162
Accredited program, information about, 16–20
ACGME. *See* Accreditation Council for Graduate Medical Education
Acronyms, 201–203
Admitting patients, 114–120
  guidelines for, 112–114
  infection control and, 112
  patient history in, 114–117
  physical examination in, 117
Advanced degree, 32–33
Advanced directive, 114
Advanced program, 52
Adverse patient care outcome, 131
Affinity credit card, 192
Aggressiveness, 72
Agreement, match participation, 53
Airway management simulation, 157
Alcohol, driving and, 194
Alert, journal, 151–152
Allergy, patient history of, 116
Allied health personnel
  listing of, 98
  relationships with, 108–110

American Board of Medical Specialties, 5
American College of Pediatrics, clinical skills workshops of, 14
American culture, 97–98
American Medical Association (AMA)
  access to information from FREIDA, 17
  Council on Medical Education of, 141
  Ethical Force Program of, 87
  information sources of, 19–20
  Virtual Mentor of, 72, 75
American medical culture, 90–94
  in general, 90–91
  mission of medical education and, 91–92
  role of residents in, 92–93
American medical system, 135–169. *See also* Medical system, American
American Osteopathic Association, 6
Anesthesia incident, 156–157
Applicant information service, ECFMG, 12
Application process
  for employment authorization, 198
  for externships and observerships, 27–33
    core competencies needed for, 29–31
    guidelines for, 28–29
  for residency program
    advanced degrees and, 32–33
    application and match cycle of, 44
    automatic uploading of documents in, 50
    California application status letter and, 49

Application process (*cont'd.*)
    credential verification in, 15–16
    curriculum vitae in, 33–35
    dean's letter for, 36–38
    document tracking system in, 50
    ECFMG certification in, 12–13
    ECFMG status report in, 49–50
    Electronic Residency Application Service in, 42–51
    interviewing in, 39–42
    letters of recommendation in, 38–39, 45–48
    marketing oneself in, 33–38
    medical school transcript in, 49
    Medical Student Performance Evaluation and, 48
    networking in, 31–32
    NRMP match in, 51–56
    on-line, 50–51
    original document policy and, 46–47
    personal statement in, 36
    photograph in, 49
    repeat, 50
    requirements for, 12–16
    for residency program, 36–38
    resources for finding, 28
    resume for, 35–36
    return of document service in, 50
    schedule for applications, 45
    supporting documents for, 44
    USMLE examinations in, 13–15
    USMLE transcript in, 49
  for social security card, 190
  for visa, 59
  visibility and, 32
Assessment, 177–181
  in admission examination, 117
  of communication skills, 81–84

Assessment (*cont'd.*)
data sources for, 177
instruments for, 178–180
self-, 174–175
Assistance, emergency, 199
Assistant, physician, 98
Assistant program director, 135–136
Association of American Medical
Colleges (AAMC)
externships and, 28
on medical student performance
evaluation, 37–38
on teamwork, 163
Attending physician
definition of, 4
malpractice and, 131
at top of hierarchy, 90
trainee's relationship with,
106–107
Attending teaching rounds, 145
Automatic uploading of document,
50
Autonomy, 160

B
B-1 visa, 59
B-2 visa, 59
Back-channel clue, 79
Bank account, 191–192
Basic requisites, 4
Behaviors, taboo, 81
Bill of Rights, Patient's, 99, 216–218
Board
of medical specialties, 5
specialty, 19
Board review conference, 146
Body odor, 81
Bulletin of Information, USMLE, 12
Business degree, 33
Buying car, 194
Buying house, 189

C
California application status letter,
49
Cambridge International English
Language Testing Service,
84
Car, buying of, 194
Card, health tips Information, 103

Career path, 8–9
Case manager, 98, 109
Case presentation, 120–121
Categorical program, 52
Centers for Medicare and Medicaid
Services, 138
Certificate, controlled substance
registration, 185–186
Certification
ECFMG, 12–13, 14
information in Green Book
about, 19
J-1 sponsorship and, 60–61
medical specialty, 186
Chairman's rounds, 145
Charity care, 140
Chart stimulated recall
examination, 178–179
Checklist for evaluation, 179
Chief complaint, 115
Child, school for, 198
Chinese surnames, 75
Citizenship and Immigration
Services, 58, 60
Claims-made insurance, 132
Clerk, ward, 98, 110
Clinical case simulations, 15
Clinical examination, 179
objective structured, 82
Clinical nutritionist, 98
Clinical psychologist, 109
Clinical Skills Evaluation
Collaboration, 13
Clinical teaching, as obligation,
4–6
Clinical trial, 154
ClinicalTrials.gov, 153
Clue, back-channel, 79
Code status, 113
Cohort study, 154
Collegiality, 164
Commitment, in microskills model,
147–148
Committee, residency review, 6,
141
Common application form, 50
Communication, 30, 71–88
about errors, 164
assessment of, 82–84
in clinical settings, 72–76

Communication (*cont'd.*)
with health care team
members, 75–76
medicalese and, 73
with patients, 73–75
writing as, 76
as core competency, 142, 143
culture and, 71–72
in educational settings, 76–77
English proficiency and, 82–84
improvement of, 84–87
in medical encounters, 104
nonverbal, 78–82
post-interview, 41–42
in social settings, 77–78
taboo behaviors, 82
with team members, 121
Community-based university-
affiliated program, 21
Competency
core, 6, 29–31, 141–143
cultural, 164
teamwork as, 162
Comprehension, 86
Conference
board review, 146
core curriculum, 146
journal club, 145
morbidity and mortality, 145–146
Confidence interval, 155
Confidentiality, 102–103, 158–159
Conflict, 72
Consent, informed, 159–160
Consultant, relationship with, 108
Consultation, protocol for, 122–123
Contract, termination of, 64
Controlled Substance Registration
Certificate, 185–186
Conversation, 78
with patient, 101–102
Core competencies, 6, 29–31,
141–143
Core curriculum conference, 146
Correction of mistakes, 149–150
Cost of care, 136–140
Counselor, financial, 98, 109
Credentials, verification of, 15, 185
Credit card, 192
Credit history, 193
Credit union, 193

Criteria for training programs, 16
Cultural competence, 164
Cultural diversity, 86–87
Culture
   American, 97–98
   language and, 71–72
   popular, 188–199. *See also*
      Popular culture
Curriculum conference, core, 146
Curriculum vitae, 33–35
   for state medical board, 184–185

D

Daily work activities, 111–128
   admitting patients, 112–117
   communication with team
      members as, 121–122
   consultation as, 122–123
   discharge planning as, 123–125
   in emergency department, 112
   follow-up and sign-out rounds,
      123
   laboratory and imaging studies,
      122
   medication reconciliation as, 125
   patient education as, 125–126
   patient management, 118–120
   presentation as, 120–121
   progress notes as, 121
   responsibilities in, 112
   typical schedule for, 111
Data collection, 118
Data of physical examination, 117
Database, library, 151
Dean's letter, 36–38, 48
Death
   as failure, 97–98
   possible malpractice in, 131
Decision, in microskills model,
   147–148
Decision-making, patient's role in,
   101–102
Defensive medicine, 130
Degree, advanced, 32–33
360-degree evaluation, 178
Department of Homeland Security,
   58
Department of State, 58
Deposition in malpractice suit,
   131

Design, study, 154
Designated institutional official,
   135
Diagnostic interview, 74
Diagnostic test, 154
Didactic session, 145–146
Diet, 193–194
Dignity, human, 100
Direct inpatient care, supervised,
   144–145
Disagreement, respectful
   expression of, 164
Discharge planning, 123–125
Disease-specific patient education,
   125
Dishonesty, academic, 77
Dismissal, 182–183
Disruptive patient, 106
Doctor of osteopathy, 6
Doctor-patient relationship. *See*
   Physician-patient
   relationship
Document
   automatic uploading of, 50
   for Electronic Residency
      Application Service, 44–51
   original, 46–47
Document submission form, 44
Document tracking system, OASIS,
   50
Documentation
   in admitting history, 114
   in clinical setting, 76
   for visit to US, 59
Dormitory, 188
Dress
   appropriate, 81
   for interview, 40
Dreyfus model of skill acquisition,
   141
Driver's license, 190–191
Driving, 194
   under influence of alcohol, 194
Drug company, research sponsored
   by, 155–156
Drug Enforcement Agency
   Controlled Substance
   Registrstion Certificate,
   185–186
Duty hours, 143–144

Dynamic List of Unfilled Positions,
   54

E

ECFMG. *See* Educational
   Commission for Foreign
   Medical Graduates
ECFMG certification, 12–13
ECFMG IMG Advisors Network
   (IAN), 210-212
ECFMG standard certificate, 14
ECFMG status report, 49–50
Education
   as mission, 92
   patient, 102, 103
Educational Commission for
   Foreign Medical Graduates,
   7, 12–13
   advisors network of, 210–212
   J-1 sponsorship and, 60–62
   resources of, 209
   spoken English proficiency
      requirement, 82–83
   status report, 49–50
Educational process, 144–166
   environment of, 144–146
      didactic sessions in, 145–146
      supervised direct inpatient
         care in, 144–145
   microskills model in, 147–150
   professionalism and ethical
      issues in, 158–161
      confidentiality and, 158–159
      informed consent and,
         159–160
      respect, autonomy, and self-
         determination and, 160–161
   residents as teachers in, 146
   resources for learning in,
      151–158
      electronic and print, 151–152
      evaluation of, 153–155
      MEDLINE database as,
         152–153
      pharmaceutical company
         sponsored research as,
         155–156
      reference management and,
         153
      simulation in, 156–158

Educational process (*cont'd.*)
  self-directed learning in, 150
  team system in, 161–166
    challenges of, 161–163
    effective, 164
    graduated levels of
      responsibility and, 163
    self-study and, 165–166
    teaching responsibilities in,
      163–165
Educational setting,
    communication in, 76–77
Electronic Residency Application
    Service (ERAS), 42–51
  application and match cycle of,
    44
  documents needed for, 44–51
  overview of, 42–43
Electronic resources, 151–152
Emergency assistance, 199
Emergency Medical Treatment and
    Active Labor Act, 139
Employee, as role of resident, 93
Employee identification number,
    federal, 186
Employment, for spouse, 198
EndNote, 153
End-of-rotation evaluation,
    181–182
English, varieties of, 85
English as second language, test
    of, 14, 83–84
English proficiency, 82–84
  self-assessment of, 83–84
ERAS. *See* Electronic Residency
    Application Service
Error
  correction of, 149–150
  open communication about,
    164
Ethical Force Program, 87
Ethical issues, 158–161
  confidentiality and, 158–159
  as core competency, 30–31
  informed consent and, 159–160
  respect, autonomy, and self-
    determination and, 160–161
Ethical responsibility, of attending
    physician, 4
Ethnic medical societies, 213–215

Evaluation, 176–183
  assessment in, 177–181
  end-of-rotation, 181–182
  feedback vs, 176–177
  medical student performance,
    37–38
  of resident, 6
  RIME, 180–181
  steps in, 177
Evidence, supporting, 148
Examination
  chart stimulated recall, 178–179
  clinical, 179
  in-training, 6, 180
  licensing, 12, 13–15
  objective structured clinical, 82
  physical, 117
  physician's demeanor during,
    104
  USMLE step, 14–15
  written, 180
Exchange Visitor Program, 60–62
External moonlighting, 129
Externship and observership,
    27–33
  advanced degrees and, 32–33
  core competencies and, 29–31
  guidelines for starting, 28–29
  networking and, 31–32
  overview of, 27
  resources for finding, 28
  visibility and, 32
Eye contact, 79–80

F

F-1 visa, moonlighting and, 129
Failure, death as, 97–98
FAIMER, 12–13
Family
  physician's relationship with,
    105–106
  of resident, 197–198
Family history, 116
Federal employee identification
    number, 186
Federation of State Medical
    Boards, 185
Feedback, 79, 172–176
  barriers to, 176
  better, 173–174

Feedback (*cont'd.*)
  evaluation vs, 176–177
  formative, 172
  positive and negative, 175–176
  problems with, 173
  sandwich, 175-176
  summative, 173
Fellow, research, 33
Fellowship and Residency
    Electronic Interactive
    Database Access (FREIDA),
    16–19
Fellowship training, 5
Female patient, observer during
    examination of, 101
Financial counselor, 98, 109
Financial issues, 136–140
  Emergency Medical Treatment
    and Active Labor Act, 139
  Medicaid, 138
  Medicare, 137–138
  uninsured patients, 139–140
  Veterans Administration, 139
First and last names, 75
First impression, 81–82
Float system, on-call, 127
Follow-up rounds, 123
Food, obtaining, 193–194
Form
  of address, 74–75
  common application, 50
  document submission, 44
Form I-765, 198
Formal and informal language, 72
Format, SOAP, 120–121
Formative feedback, 172
Foundation of the Advancement of
    International Medical
    Education and Research
    (FAIMER), 12–13
Fraudulent letter of
    recommendation, 39
Freedom, 99
FREIDA online, 16–19
Frontier spirit, 97–98
Funding of medical care, 136–140

G

Gallows humor, 91
General rules, teaching of, 148–149

Gestures, 80
Glossary, 201-203
Goals of team, 164
Google Scholar, 153
Government oversight of visas, 58
Graduate Medical Education
        Directory, 17, 18–19
Graduate medical education
        training
    international, 7–8
    osteopathic, 6
    requisites for, 4
    structure and length of, 4
    teaching responsibilities in, 4–6
Graduate program Web site, 20
Green Book, 17, 18–19
Green card status, 9
Greeting of patient, 101–102
Grocery shopping, 193–194
Group activities, 196–197

H
H-4 visa, 62
Handshake, 81, 101
H-1B visa, 9, 60
    moonlighting and, 130
    for training, 62–63
Health care, personal, 195
Health care system, 135–169. *See
        also* Medical system,
        American
Health care team. *See* Team
Health Insurance Portability and
        Accountability Act (HIPAA),
        102
Health literacy, 102
Health tips Information card, 103
Hierarchy in medicine, 90
High-fidelity patient care model,
        157
HIPAA, 102
History
    admission, 114–117
    credit, 193
Home care, assessing need for, 123
Hospital dormitory, 188
Hospitalist physician, 108
House, buying of, 189
H&P (admission history and
        physical), 114–117

Human dignity, 100
Humor, gallows, 91

I
Identification number
    federal employee, 186
    USMLE/ECFMG, 12
Imaging, 122
IMED, 12–13
Immigration, 58–65
    travel outside U.S. and, 65
    visa for, 58–65
Immigration status, 8–9
*Improving Communication - Improving
        Care*, 87
Incident, anesthesia, 156–157
Independence, 99
Infection control, 113
Information
    of accredited program, 16–20
    local, 199
    patient's understanding of, 102
Information booklet, ECFMG, 12
Information card for patient, 103
Informed consent, 159–160
Initial entry to United States, 65
Institution
    information in Green Book
        about, 19
    residency review committee of,
        6
    in selecting specialty, 21
Instrument, assessment, 178–180
Insurance
    malpractice, 132
    uninsured patient and, 139–140
Insurance provider number, 185
Integrity of research, 167
Internal moonlighting, 128
International graduate medical
        education training
    career paths after, 8–9
    trends in, 7–8
International Medical Education
        Directory, 12–13
Internet Web sites, 204-207
Interpersonal skills, 30, 83
    as core competency, 142, 143
Interruption, 78
Interval, confidence, 155

Interview
    diagnostic, 74
    for residency position, 39–42
In-training examination, 6, 180

J
J-1 sponsorship for training, 60–62
J-1 visa, 8–9, 60
    moonlighting and, 129–130
J-2 visa, 60
Journal, medical, 151–152
Journal club, 145
Junior resident
    relationship with senior resident,
        107–108
    teaching of, 165

L
Labor, dignity of, 100
Laboratory study, 122
Language. *See also* Communication
    cultural diversity and, 86–87
    and culture, 71–72
    testing proficiency of, 13–14
Language and speech pathologist,
        98, 110
Leadership, sharing of, 164
Learning, 4–6
    practice-based, 30, 142, 143
    self-directed, 150
    in team system, 161–166
Learning resources, 151–158
Legal issues
    of J-1 visa holder, 61
    malpractice as, 130–132
Legal responsibility of attending
        physician, 4, 106–107
Letter
    California application status, 49
    dean's, 36–38, 48
    of recommendation, 38–39,
        45–46
    fraudulent, 47–48
    waiver of rights to see, 47
Liaison, training program, 62
Library, medical, 151–158
License
    driver's, 190–191
    graduate medication education
        and, 5

Licensed practical nurse, 98
  relationship with, 108
Licensing examination, 12
  practical advice about, 13–14
  preparation for, 14
  standard certificate of, 14
  step 3, 15
Licensure, 183–184
  information in Green Book
    about, 19
Likelihood ratio, 154–155
List, rank order, 52–53
Listening, 86, 164
Literacy, health, 102
Literature, medical, 152–153
  critical evaluation of, 153–154
Local information, 199
Location of program, 22
Log in evaluation, 179

M

Macro level of health care, 31
Maintenance of certification
    program, 5
Malpractice, 130–132
Malpractice insurance, 132
Management
  patient, 118–120
  risk, 106
Management plan, 97
Manager, case, 98, 109
Marketing oneself, 33–42
  curriculum vitae for, 33–35
  resume for, 35–36
Master's degree, 33
Match participation agreement, 53
Matching program, NRMP, 51–56.
    See also National Resident
    Matching Program
MD/MBA degree, 33
Medicaid, 138
Medical culture, American, 90–94
  in general, 90–91
  mission of medical education
    and, 91–92
  role of residents in, 92–93
Medical history, 114–117
Medical knowledge as core
    competency, 29, 142, 143
Medical library, 151–158

Medical license, 12, 13–14, 19,
    183–184
Medical literature, 152–153
  critical evaluation of, 153–154
Medical malpractice, 130–132
Medical school transcript, 49
Medical societies, ethnic, 213–215
Medical specialty, 20–21
  certification, 186
Medical student
  performance evaluation of,
    37–38, 48
  teaching of, 121, 164–165
Medical Subject Headings index,
    152
Medical system, American, 135–169
  Accreditation Council for
    Graduate Medical Education
    and, 140–144
    core competencies and,
      141–143
    duty hours, 143–144
    overview of, 140–141
  administrative structure of, 135
  educational process of, 144–166.
    See also Educational process
  financial issues in, 136–140
    Emergency Medical Treatment
      and Active Labor Act, 139
    Medicaid, 138
    Medicare, 137–138
    uninsured patients, 139–140
    Veterans Administration, 139
  research opportunities in,
    166–169
  safety net in, 140
Medicalese, 73
Medicare, 137–138
Medication
  patient education about,
    125–126
  patient history of, 116
  patient's list of, 113
Medication reconciliation, 125
Medicine, defensive, 130
MEDLINE, 152–153
Meeting with patient's family,
    105–106
Mentoring, sharing of, 164
MeSH index, 152

Metaphors, common, 78
Micro level of health care, 31
Microskills model, 147–150
Military-based program, 21–22
Misconduct, research, 167
Mission of medical education,
    91–92
Mistakes, correction of, 149–150
Model
  Dreyfus, of skill acquisition, 141
  in evaluation, 180
  high-fidelity patient care, 157
  microskills, 147–150
Monitoring, of moonlighting, 129
Moonlighting, 128–130
Morbidity and mortality
    conference, 145–146
Morning report, 145
Mortality and morbidity
    conference, 145–146
MPH degree, 33
Multidisciplinary team, 161–166
My NCBI, 153

N

Name, first and last, 75
National Board of Medical
    Examiners, 14
National Institutes of Health,
    funding of research by, 167
National Library of Medicine, 152
National Resident Matching
    Program (NRMP), 51–56
  international medical graduates
    and, 23
  participation in, 51–52
  positions outside of, 55–56
  purpose of, 51
  rank order list in, 52–53
  San Francisco match and, 55
  sequence of, 53–55
Needs, human, 100
Networking, 31–32
New patient, 118–119
Night float system, 127
Nonverbal communication, 78–82
  back-channel clues of, 79
  eye contact and, 79–80
  first impressions and, 81
  gestures as, 80

Nonverbal communication (*cont'd.*)
   personal space and, 79
   taboo behaviors, 82
   touch as, 80
Note, thank-you, 41–42
Notes, daily, 121
NRMP, 51–56. *See also* National
      Resident Matching Program
Number
   federal employee identification,
      186
   identification, USMLE/ECFMG,
      12
   insurance provider, 185
Nurse
   licensed practical, 98
   registered, 98
   role of, 75–76
   specialty, 98
Nurse practitioner, 108
Nurse-physician relationship,
    108
Nursing Relief for Disadvantaged
    Areas Act, 139
Nutritionist, clinical, 98

O
O-1 visa, 60
OASIS document tracking system,
    50
Objective clinical examination,
    179
Objective structured clinical
    examination, 82
Observer during examination,
    101
Observership, 27–33. *See also*
    Externship and observership
Obsession with time, 98
Occupational therapist, 98, 109
Odor, body, 81
Office of graduate medical
    education, 135
On-call, 126–128
   restrictions on, 143–144
One-minute preceptor, 147–150
Online information, 16–20
Optional training visa, 33
Organizational sponsor, 135
Original document policy, 46–47

Osteopathic graduate medical
    education, 6
Out of court settlement, 131–132

P
Paperwork, regulatory, 184–186
Participation agreement, match, 53
Past medical history, 114–117
Patient
   admission of, 112–114
     history and physical and,
      114–117
   communicating with, 73–75
   disruptive, 106
   medications taken by, 113
   relationship with physician,
     100–105
   respect for, 73, 160
   standardized, 157
   talking about, 76
   uninsured, 139–140
Patient care, 5–6, 95–132
   attending-trainee relationship in,
     106–107
   as core competency, 29, 141, 142
   daily work activities in, 111–128.
     See also Daily work activities
   malpractice and, 130–132
   as mission of medical education,
     91
   on-call, 126–128
   physician-patient relationship in,
     73–75, 100–105
   relationship with family in,
     105–106
   responsibility for, 163
   supervised direct, 144–145
   supervised training and, 97
   working outside residency
     program, 128–130
Patient education, 125
Patient management, 118–120
Patient survey, 179
Patient's Bill of Rights, 99, 216–218
Payment system for care, 100,
    136–140
Performance evaluation, 37–38
Permanent resident status, 9
Personal health care, 195
Personal space, 79, 99

Personal statement, 36, 37, 51
Persuasion, restrictions on, 54
Pharmaceutical company, research
    sponsored by, 155–156
Phlebotomist, 91
Photograph of applicant, 49
Physical, admission, 114–117
Physical examination, 117
Physical therapist, 98, 109
Physician
   attending
     definition of, 4
     malpractice and, 131
     at top of hierarchy, 90
     trainee's relationship with,
      106–107
   demeanor during examination,
     104
   hospitalist, 108
   role of, 92
Physician assistant, 98
   relationship with, 108
Physician-family relationship, 105
Physician-nurse relationship, 108
Physician-patient relationship
   communication in, 73–75
   confidentiality in, 102–103
   disclosure of bad news in,
     104–105
   greeting and conversation in,
     101–102
   physician's demeanor in, 104
Plagiarism, 77
Plan
   discharge, 123–124
   management, 97
Planning, discharge, 123–125
Policy, original document, 46–47
Popular culture, 188–199
   bank accounts and, 191–192
   credit cards and, 192–193
   driver's license and, 190–191
   emergency assistance and, 199
   family considerations and,
     197–198
   finding living quarters, 188–189
   food and, 193–194
   getting local information and,
     199
   personal health care and, 195

Popular culture (cont'd.)
  recreational activities and,
    196–197
  religious activities and, 195
  social security card and, 189–190
  transportation and, 194–195
Portfolio, 179
Positive reinforcement, 149
Post-interview communication,
    41–42
Power of attorney, 113–114
Practical nurse, licensed, 98
  relationship with, 108
Practice, system-based, 31
Practice-based learning, 30, 142,
    143
Preceptor, one-minute, 147–150
Preliminary program, 53
Present illness, history of, 115
Presentation
  clinical, 77
  for teaching rounds, 120–121
Presentation of case, 120–121
Pretest probability, 155
Print resources, 151–152
Private school, 198
Probability, pretest, 155
Professional networking, 31–32
Professionalism, 142, 143, 158–161
  confidentiality and, 158–159
  as core competency, 30–31
  informed consent and, 159–160
  respect, autonomy, and self-
    determination and, 160–161
Proficiency, English, 82–84
Program director, 135–136
Progress notes, 121
Promotion, 182
Protocol, sign-out, 127
Psychologist, clinical, 109
Public health, 139–140
Public school, 198
Public transportation, 194–195
PubMed search, 152
Punctuality, importance of, 90

Q

Questions
  in application interview, 40–41
  in diagnostic interview, 74

R

Radiology technologist, 98, 109
Randomized controlled trials, 154
Rank order list, 52–53
Ratio, likelihood, 154–155
Recall examination, chart
    stimulated, 178–179
Recommendation letter, 45–46
Reconciliation, medication, 125
Recreational activities, 196–197
References
  list of, 208
  management of, 153
Reflection, 176
Registered nurse, relationship with,
    108
Registered nurse, 98
Registration certificate, controlled
    substance, 185–186
Regulatory paperwork, 184–186
Reinforcement, positive, 149
Relationship
  among hospital staff, 99
  nurse-physician, 108
  physician-patient,
    communication in, 73–75
  principles of, 100–101
  with team members and trainee,
    107–108
  trainee-attending physician,
    106–107
Relationships, in team, 164
Religious activities, 195
Rental property, 188–189
Report
  ECFMG status, 49–50
  morning, 145
Request for letter of
    recommendation, 39
Requirement
  spoken English proficiency, 82–83
  for visa application, 59
Requisites, basic, 4
Research, 166–169
  funding of, 167
  integrity of, 167–168
  involvement in, 166–167
  misconduct concerning, 167
  participation in, 167–168
  types of, 154–156

Research career, 33
Residency, 12. See also Resident
  application requirements for,
    12–16
    credential verification in,
      15–16
    ECFMG certification, 12–13
    transcripts and, 15–16
    USMLE examinations, 13–15
  information sources for, 16–20
    FREIDA, 16–20
    graduate medical education
      directory, 18–19
    other sources, 19–20
  overview of, 4–9
  selection of specialty, 20–23
  working outside of, 128–130
Residency review committee, 6, 141
Resident. See also Residency
  family concerns of, 197–198
  junior
    senior resident and, 107–108
    teaching of, 165
  research by, 166–169
  role of, 92–93
  senior
    relationship with trainee,
      107–108
    work rounds and, 119–120
  as teacher, 146
Resources
  ECFMG, 209
  for communication problems,
    85–86
  for conflict resolution, 72
  for finding externships, 28
  on FREIDA, 17–18
  for learning, 151–158
    electronic and print, 151–152
    evaluation of, 153–155
    MEDLINE database as,
      152–153
    pharmaceutical company
      sponsored research as,
      155–156
    reference management and,
      153
    simulation in, 156–158
Respect for patient, 72, 160
Respiratory therapist, 98, 110

Responsibility
  of attending physician, 4,
      106–107
  graduated levels of, 163
  malpractice and, 131
  patients', 99
  for teaching, 163–165
  when on-call, 127–128
Resume, 35–36
Resuscitation simulation, 157
Retention, 182
Return of document service, 50
Review conference, board, 146
Review of systems, 117
RIME evaluation system, 180–181
Risk management, 106
Role
  of nurse, 75–76
  patient's, in decision-making,
      101–102
Rounds, 5
  attending teaching, 145
  chairman's, 145
  follow-up, 123
  sign-out, 123
  teaching, guidelines for,
      120–121
  work, 119, 145
Rules, general, 148–149

S

Safety net health care system, 140
San Francisco match, 55
Schedule
  duty hours, 143–144
  for ERAS application, 45
  on-call, 126–127
School, enrolling children in, 198
Scientific integrity, 167
Scut work, 91
Search, PubMed, 152
Secretary, ward, 98, 110
Selection of specialty, 20–23
Self-assessment, 174–175
  of English proficiency, 83–84
Self-awareness, 164
Self-determination, 160–161
Self-directed learning, 150
Self-representation, 72
Self-study, 165–166

Senior resident
  relationship with trainee,
      107–108
  work rounds and, 119–120
Seniority, 100
Sensitivity of diagnostic test,
      154–155
SEVIS, 61. *See also* Student
      Exchange Visitor
      Information System
Sexual history, 116–117
Sign-out protocol, 127
Sign-out rounds, 123
Simulated patient for clinical
      examination, 82
Simulation, 156–158
  clinical case, 15
  in evaluation, 180
Skill
  communication, 71–88. *See also*
      Communication
  human relations, 100
  interpersonal, 83
Skill acquisition, Dreyfus model of,
      141
Small-talk, 77–78
Smells, body, 81
SOAP format, 120–121
Social history, 116
Social Security Act, Medicaid
      established through, 138
Social security card, 189–190
Social setting, communication in,
      77–78
Social worker, 98, 110
Society, medical, 213–215
Space, personal, 79, 99
Spanish surnames, 75
Specialty
  changing of, 62
  listing in Green Book, 19
  medical or surgical, 20–21
  selection of, 20–23
Specialty nurse, 98
Specialty training, 4
Specificity of diagnostic test,
      154–155
Speech and language pathologist,
      98, 110
Spoken English proficiency, 82–84

Spoken English proficiency
      examination, 13–14
Sponsor, organizational, 135
Sponsoring organization, 135
Sponsorship, J-1, 60–62
Spouse of resident, 197–198
Standard certificate, ECFMG, 14
Standard duties when on-call,
      127–128
Standardized patient, 157
Standardized patient for clinical
      examination, 82
Statement, personal, 51
Status letter, California application,
      49
Status report, ECFMG, 49–50
Step examinations, USMLE, 14–15
Structured clinical examination,
      objective, 82
Student Exchange Visitor
      Information System, 61
Study
  laboratory, 122
  self-, 165–166
Subspecialty training, 4, 5
Summary, discharge, 124–125
Summative feedback, 173
Superspecialty, 4, 5
Supervised direct inpatient care,
      144–145
Support services, ERAS, 48
Supporting evidence, 148
Surgical specialty, 20–21
Surname, 75
Survey, patient, 179
System-based practice, as core
      competency, 31
Systems-based practice, 142, 143

T

Taboo behaviors, 81
Task trainer, 157
Tattoo, 81
Teacher, resident as, 146
Teaching
  of general rules, 148–149
  of medical students, 121
  obligation for, 4–6
  responsibility for, 163–165
  as role of resident, 93

Teaching institution, 19
Teaching rounds
    attending, 145
    guidelines for, 120–121
Team, health care
    communication with, 75–76
    effective, 164
    learning within, 161–166
    relationship with trainee,
        107–108
Team system
    challenges of, 161–163
    effective, 164
    graduated levels of responsibility
        and, 163
    self-study and, 165–166
    teaching responsibilities in,
        163–165
Teamwork, 90–91
Technologist, radiology, 98, 109
Temporary worker visa, 60
    for GME training, 61–62
Termination of contract, 64
Test
    diagnostic, 154
    of English as Foreign Language,
        14, 83–84
    of English for International
        Communication, 84
Thank-you note, 41–42
Therapist
    occupational, 98, 109
    physical, 98, 109
    respiratory, 98, 110
Thomas Prometric Testing Services,
    15
360-degree evaluation, 178
Time, American obsession with, 98
Touch, 80, 90
Tracking system, OASIS document,
    50
Trainee, attending physician's
    relationship with, 106–107

Training, fellowship, 5
Training program liaison, 62, 135,
    136
Transcript
    medical school, 49
    USMLE, 49
    verification of, 15
Transfer, request for, 64
Transitioning to United States,
    58–66
    initial entry and, 65–66
    visa issues and, 58–65
Translation services, 87
Transportation, 194–195
Travel, 197
    outside U.S., 65
    visa for, 58–65. See also Visa
Trial, clinical, 154

U

Uninsured patient, 139–140
United States Medical Licensing
        Examination (USMLE), 12,
        13–15
University-based program, 21
Uploading of document, automatic,
    50
U.S. Citizenship and Immigration
        Services, 59, 60
USMLE step 3 examination, 15
USMLE transcript, 49
USMLE/ECFMG identification
        number, 12

V

Varieties of English, 85
Verification of credentials, 15,
    185
Veterans Administration, 21–22,
    139
Vignettes for improving
        communication skills, 84

Virtual Mentor, 72, 75
    for improving communication
        skills, 84
Visa, 58–65
    application process for, 59
    government oversight of, 58
    H-1B, 9
        documentation for, 63
        for training, 62–63
    H-4, 62
    J-1, 8–9, 60–62
        documentation for, 63
        minimum requirements for, 62
    J-2, 60
    maintaining status, 64–65
    moonlighting and, 129–130
    optional training, 33
    options for, 60
    visitor, 58–59
Visa stamp, 65
Visiting Student Application
        Service, 28
Visitor visa, 58–59

W

Waiver
    concerning letters of
        recommendation, 47
    of visa requirement, 8–9
Ward clerk, 98, 110
Web site
    ECFMG, 12
    graduate program, 20
    list of, 203–207
Work activities, daily, 111–128. See
        also Daily work activities
Work rounds, 5, 119, 145
Working hours, 143–144
Working outside residency
        program, 128–130
Workshop, clinical skills, 14
Writing, 76
Written examination, 180